AF316732

MITRAL STENOSIS

Collected Reprints
(1970-2019)

By
WILLIAM C. ROBERTS, MD
and
COLLEAGUES

ISBN: 979-8-88862-150-9
Printed in the United States of America on acid-free paper.

Preface

In the early parts of the 20th century, rheumatic mitral stenosis was a common and devastating condition. Elliott Cutler at the Peter Bent Brigham Hospital in Boston attempted in several patients mitral commissurotomy without success. It was not until 25 years later in Philadelphia that the procedure was carried out successfully. Thus, mitral commissurotomy became the first successful cardiac operation (patent ductus arteriosus and aortic isthmus coarctation are not part of the heart). Today, in the Western world, rheumatic mitral stenosis is relatively infrequent. Detailed morphologic study of the rheumatic mitral stenotic valve has disclosed that the thickening of the leaflets and chordae tendineae is due to superimposed fibrous tissue, not to intrinsic damage to the leaflets and chordae themselves. Occasionally, fibrin deposits are seen suggesting that the superimposed fibrous tissue is the result of organization of fibrin thrombi. Today in the Western world mitral stenosis is likely more commonly the result of massive mitral annular calcific deposits rather than the rheumatic process.

—William C. Roberts, MD

Table of Contents

*Articles are numbered based on WCR's CV.

Giant right atrium in rheumatic mitral stenosis

Atrial enlargement restricted by mural calcification

*William C. Roberts, M.D.**
J. O'Neal Humphries, M.D.
Andrew G. Morrow, M.D.
Bethesda and Baltimore, Md.

In most patients with rheumatic mitral stenosis or regurgitation some degree of left atrial enlargement is evident, and when the left atrium becomes greatly dilated, the right atrial chamber is usually also quite large, even though the tricuspid valve leaflets and chordae tendineae may be anatomically normal. Enormous dilatation of the right atrium with only slight and quite disproportionate enlargement of the left atrium has not been reported in patients with acquired mitral valve disease. These were the unusual findings, however, in 3 patients recently studied by us. A description of the clinical and pathologic observations in these three patients is presented in the report which follows.

Patients studied

Pertinent clinical and necropsy features in the 3 patients are summarized in Table I. All had histories of acute rheumatic fever and long-standing symptoms of cardiac dysfunction. In each mitral commissurotomy had been performed 6 to 9 years previously. Left atrial thrombi had been encountered at mitral commissurotomy in Patients Nos. 1 and 2, but none had had a systemic embolus. Before commissurotomy, Patients 1 and 2 had pure mitral stenosis; Patient No. 3, in addition to severe mitral stenosis, had a blowing systolic murmur compatible with tricuspid regurgitation, although there was no jugular venous distention, hepatomegaly, ascites, or subcutaneous edema. This patient had had this murmur at least since he was 19 years old, at which time he was suspected of having a pulmonary embolus. Angiography at that time, in addition to showing poor filling of the pulmonary arteries to the lower lobes, also showed a hugely dilated right atrium and a normal-sized left atrium. Mitral commissurotomy was performed at age 33, and a systolic thrill was palpated over the right atrium at that time.

Each of the 3 patients was improved by mitral commissurotomy, but symptoms of cardiac dysfunction recurred two (Patients 1 and 3) to nine years (Patient 2) later. Severe right-sided congestive cardiac failure with dependent subcutaneous edema, ascites, pleural effusion, a large and pulsatile liver, and progressive deterioration occurred in each patient, almost certainly the result of restenosis of the mitral valve and concomitant development or worsening of tricuspid regurgitation. Precordial murmurs typical of tricuspid regurgitation were

From the Section of Pathology and the Clinic of Surgery, National Heart Institute, Bethesda, Md., and the Division of Cardiology, Department of Medicine, The Johns Hopkins University and Hospital, Baltimore, Md.

Received for publication March 19, 1969.

*Reprint requests to: Dr. Roberts, Building 10A, Room 3E30, National Institutes of Health, Bethesda, Md. 20014.

Table I. Giant right atrium and nearly normal-sized left atrium in mitral stenosis

Patient	Age, sex	Length of symptoms (yr.)	Cardiac valvular lesions	ECG	Age at cardiac cath. (yr.)	PA	RV†	RA	LA	LV†	SA	LA-LV mean gradient	CO/CI	Heart weight (Gm.)
1, M. V. A65-36	57, F	24	MS TR*	AF RVH	57		52/15	m15 v22	m19 v29	118/12	118/61	8	4.6/3.1	680
2, E. L. A65-149	32, F	11	MS TR*	AF RVH	22	53/32	55/7	m4 v5	m17 v23		120/65		3.3/1.9	560
					29	36/20	36/4		m15 v22	96/6	116/72	5	3.5/2.0	
					32	59/41	59/17	m23 v36	m26				2.3/1.3	
3, J. S. JHH 36136	39, M	26	MS TR	AF RVH RBBB	19	73/45	73/0				125/62			850
					33	64/22	72/0	m9 v18	v28	135/6	135/65	15	3.4/2.0	
					38	82/32	83/12	m25 v35		118/8	123/79		6.0/3.5	

Abbreviations: Cath., Catheterization; PA, pulmonary artery; RV, right ventricle; RA, right atrium; LA, left atrium; LV, left ventricle; SA, systemic artery; CO, cardiac output; CI, cardiac index; MS, mitral stenosis; TR, tricuspid regurgitation; AF, atrial fibrillation; RVH, right ventricular hypertrophy; RBBB, right bundle branch block; m, mean; v, v wave.

*TR was not present before mitral commissurotomy.

†Systolic and end-diastolic pressures.

audible in each patient after the recurrence of symptoms of cardiac dysfunction. Reoperation was carried out in 2 patients; in Patient 1 the tricuspid valve was replaced, another mitral commissurotomy was performed, and a portion of the redundant right atrial wall was resected; in Patient 3 the mitral valve was replaced and a tricuspid annuloplasty performed. In both patients severe tricuspid regurgitation was evident at operation. Patient No. 2 died before reoperation was performed. Patient No. 1 died 10 days postoperatively of inadequate cardiac output, probably the result of operatively induced mitral regurgitation, and Patient No. 3 died 4 months postoperatively from consequences of prosthetic mitral stenosis resulting from interference to ball movement by the left ventricular wall.

Necropsy in each patient disclosed a large heart, an enormous right atrium, a mildly dilated left atrium, diffuse calcific deposits of the left atrial and atrial septal walls, and mitral valve leaflets, but no calcification of the right atrial walls. The tricuspid valve leaflets and chordae tendineae were thickened and fibrous in each patient. All 3 patients had extensive pulmonary vascular and parenchymal changes, and congestion of all viscera, including severe centrolobular hepatic necrosis, hemorrhage, and fibrosis. Various clinical and necropsy findings of particular interest are illustrated in Figs. 1 through 7.

Discussion

Extreme, enormous, or giant-sized dilatation of the left atrium (probably greater than 1,000 ml. capacity; normal less than 150 ml.[1,2]) has been discussed for years.[1,3-8] These reports indicate that enormous left atrial dilatation nearly always occurs in patients with mitral valvular disease. The mitral lesion may be pure regurgitation, pure stenosis, or a combination of the two, and there is some controversy as to which of these functional alterations is most frequently associated with a giant-sized left atrium. Also, the reason that one patient with mitral dysfunction has a huge left atrium and another with a similar functional abnormality has only minimal left atrial dilatation has not been resolved.

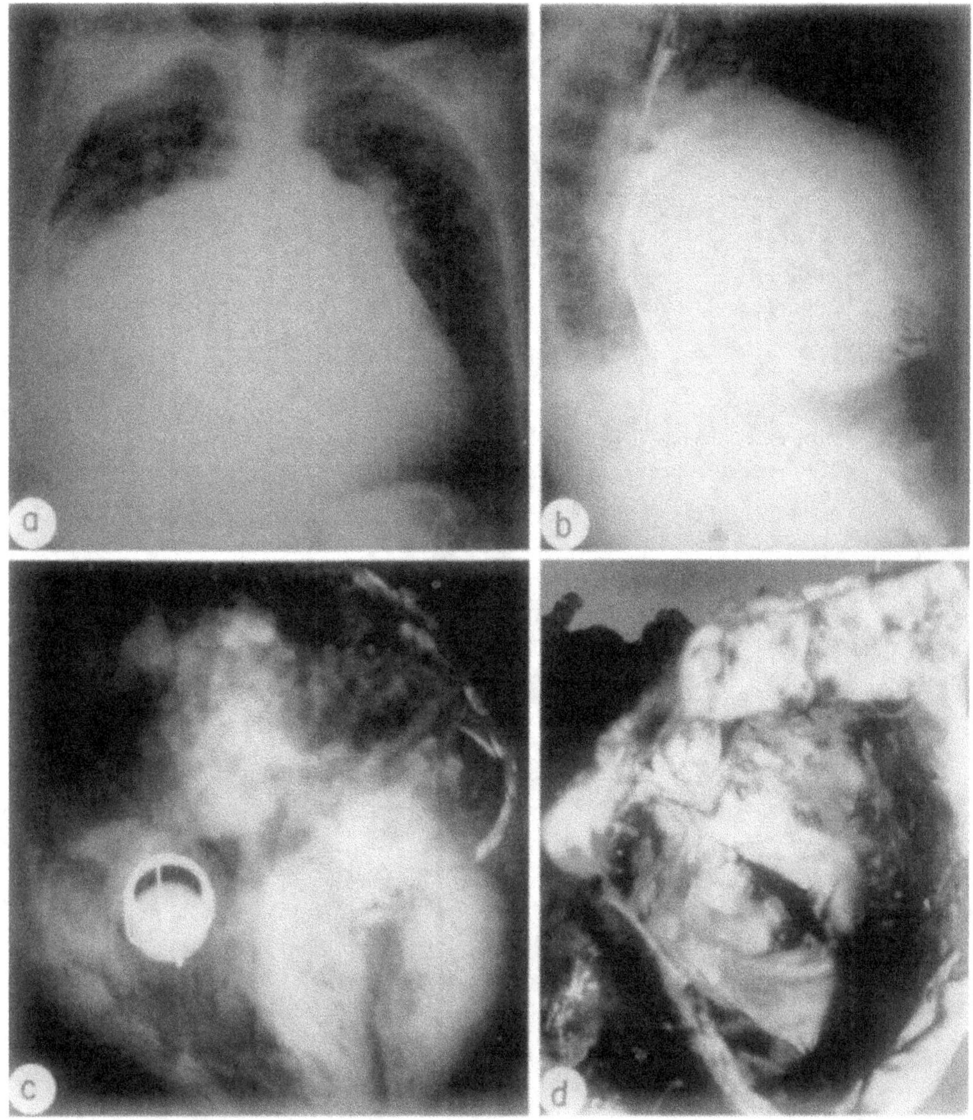

Fig. *1*. Patient 1 (Table 1). *a* and *b*, Chest roentgenograms taken 3 weeks before death. The huge right atrium forms the right border of the heart on the posteroanterior view. *c*, Radiograph of the heart specimen. The left atrial wall is calcified. Much of the right atrial wall was excised at operation. The tricuspid valve was replaced with a Starr-Edwards prosthesis, and a mitral commissurotomy was also done. *d*, Opened left atrium showign its calcified wall which also is focally covered by thrombi.

Nearly all patients with enormous left atria have histories of acute rheumatic fever or chorea, and it has been suggested that they have more severe attacks of, or more relapses of, acute rheumatic fever than do patients with similar valvular lesions and less left atrial dilatation. Since rheumatic fever always involves the left atrial wall,[9] it is reasonable to speculate that if the inflammatory process was severe or occurred repeatedly the atrial wall would be more damaged, consequently more compliant or elastic, and, therefore, more easily dilated by increased intra-atrial pressure. Although nearly all patients with chronic rheumatic mitral disease have abnormal left atrial walls, the degree of myocardial destruction and fibrosis appears to be far worse in the subjects with dilated left atria than in those with smaller sized chambers.

Patients with giant-sized left atria and

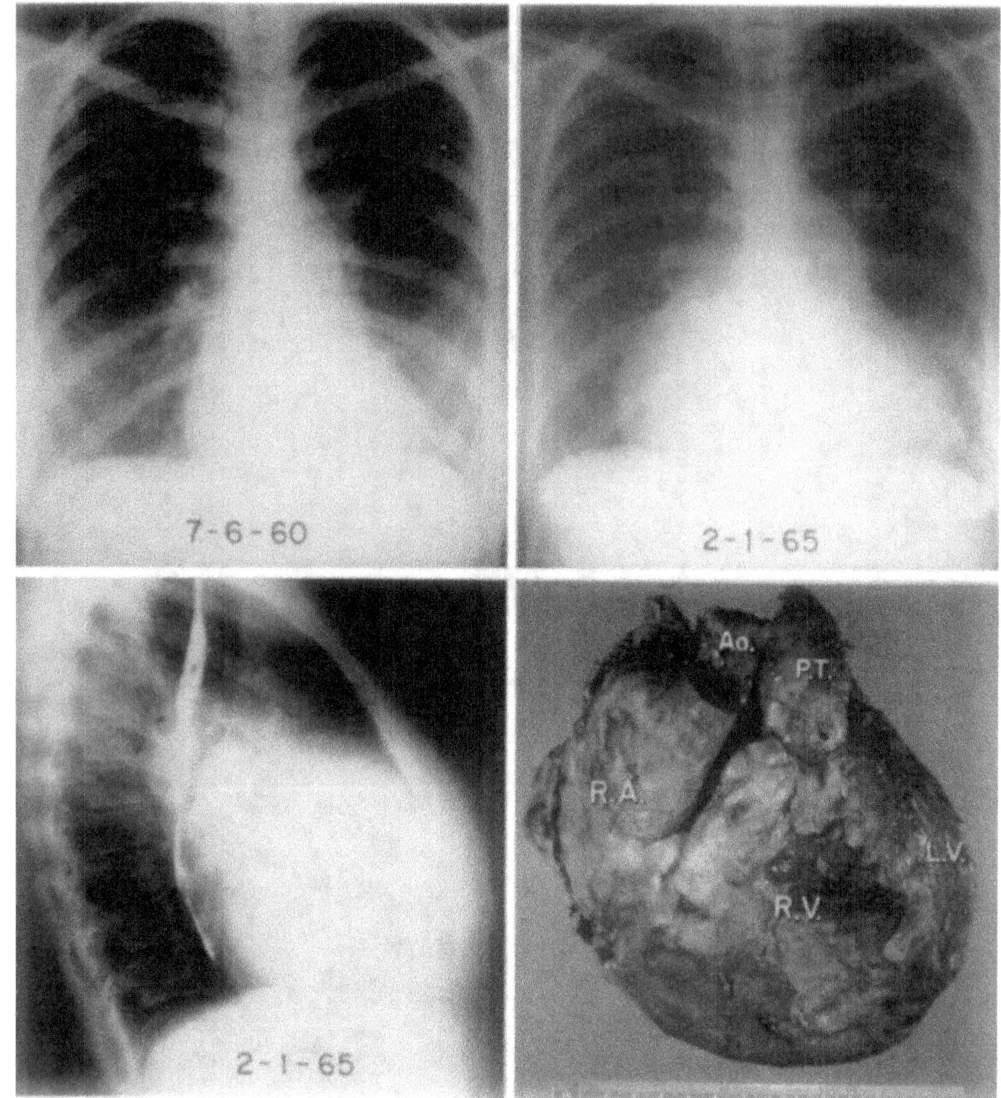

Fig. 2. Patient No. 2. *Upper* and *lower left:* Chest roentgenograms taken on the dates shown. The patient died Aug. 13, 1965. *Lower right:* Anterior surface of heart. The left atrium is not visible anteriorly but the right atrium (*R.A.*) is very large. *R.V.*, Right ventricle; *L.V.*, left ventricle; *P.T.*, pulmonary trunk; *Ao*, aorta.

severe mitral valvular disease usually have only slightly elevated or even normal left atrial, pulmonary venous, pulmonary arterial and right ventricular pressures.[10] In contrast, these pressures are usually quite high in subjects with only mildly dilated or normal-sized left atria and severe mitral valvular disease.[11] The small left atrium is less compliant, and reflects its elevated pressure to the lung and to the right ventricle, whereas the hugely dilated left atrium is readily compliant and "absorbs" the pressure energy. In most patients with giant left atrium the right atrium is also dilated, but is never as large as the left.[1,6] Right atrial dilatation occurs as the result of tricuspid regurgitation, which may be either organic or functional in type and with or without accompanying tricuspid stenosis. Stretching of the atrial septum by the dilatation of the left atrium probably contributes to the dilatation of the right atrium also.

Many reports have described the occurrence of giant left atrium in patients with mitral valvular disease, but the oc-

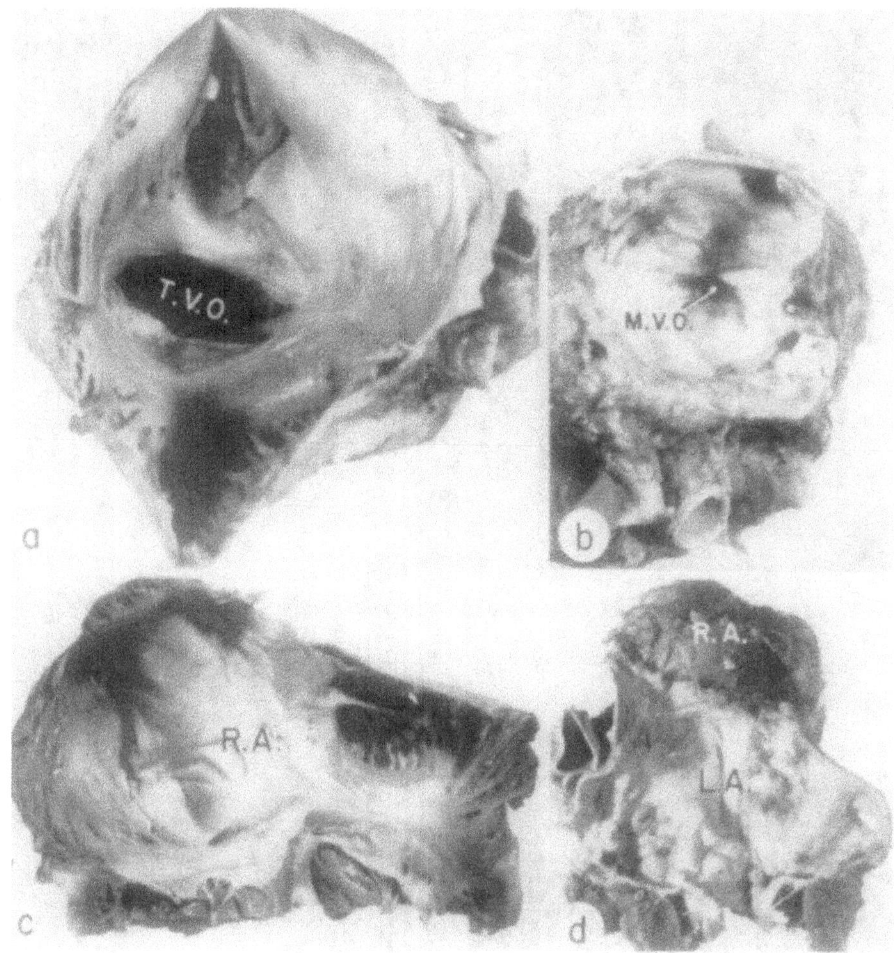

Fig. 3. Heart in Patient No. 2. *a* and *b* were photographed at the same magnification; in *a* the huge right atrium has been partially opened showing the dilated tricuspid valve orifice (*T.V.O.*), and in *b* the only slightly dilated left atrium has been partially opened showing the stenotic mitral valve orifice (*M.V.O.*). *c* and *d* likewise were taken at the same magnification and show a huge right atrium (*R.A.*) in *c* compared to an only slightly dilated left atrium (*L.A.*) in *d*. The left atrial wall contains many deposits of calcium. The tricuspid leaflets are only slightly thickened, not enough in themselves to account for the tricuspid regurgitation.

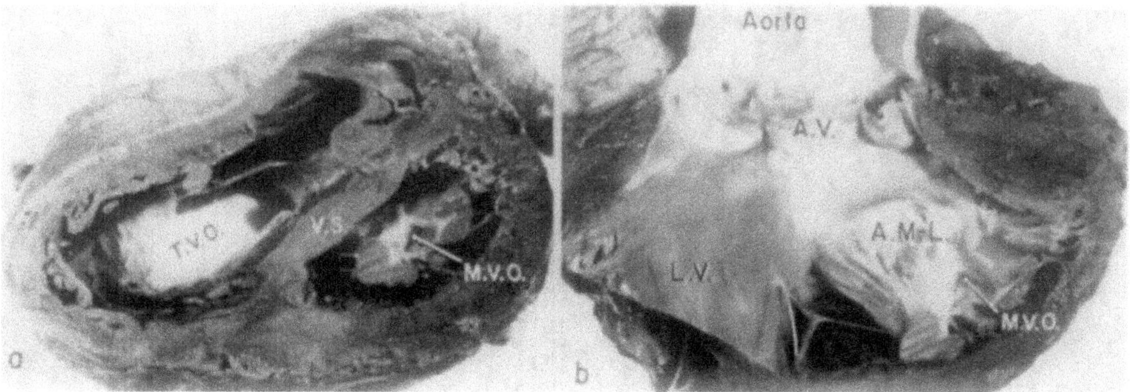

Fig. 4. Heart in Patient No. 2. *a*, The caudal portions of the ventricles have been removed. The right ventricular cavity is much larger than the left, and the mitral valve orifice (*M.V.O.*) is severely stenotic. The tricuspid valve orifice (*T.V.O.*), in contrast, is greatly dilated. *b*, Opened aorta, normal aortic valve (*A.V.*) and left ventricular outflow tract (*L.V.*). The mitral leaflets insert directly into the papillary muscles. The cause of the left ventricular dilatation is uncertain. *A.M.L.*, Anterior mitral leaflet.

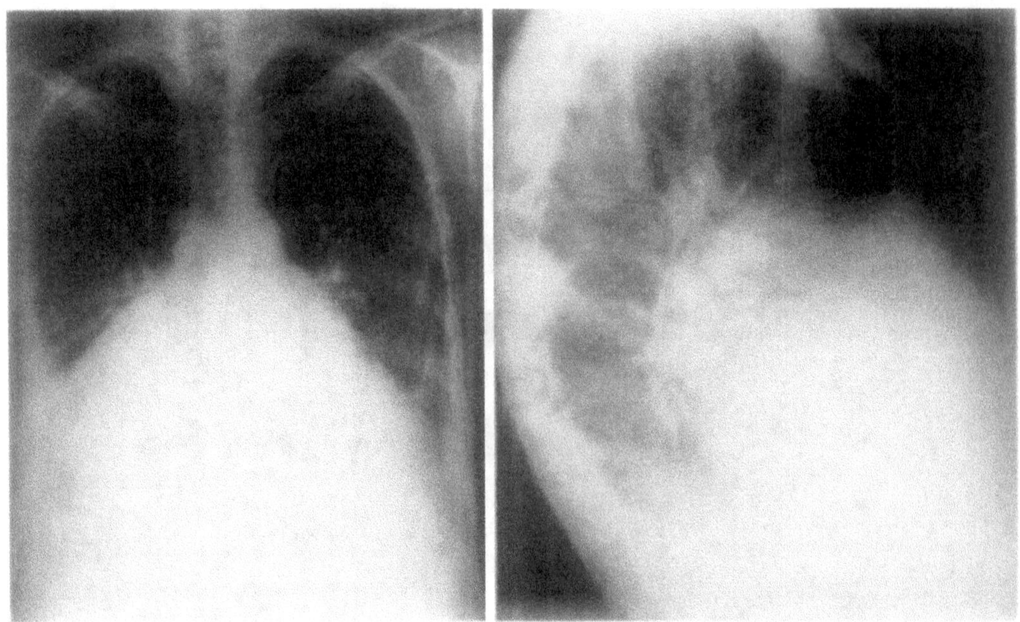

Fig. 5. Chest roentgenograms in Patient No. 3 taken 5 months before death.

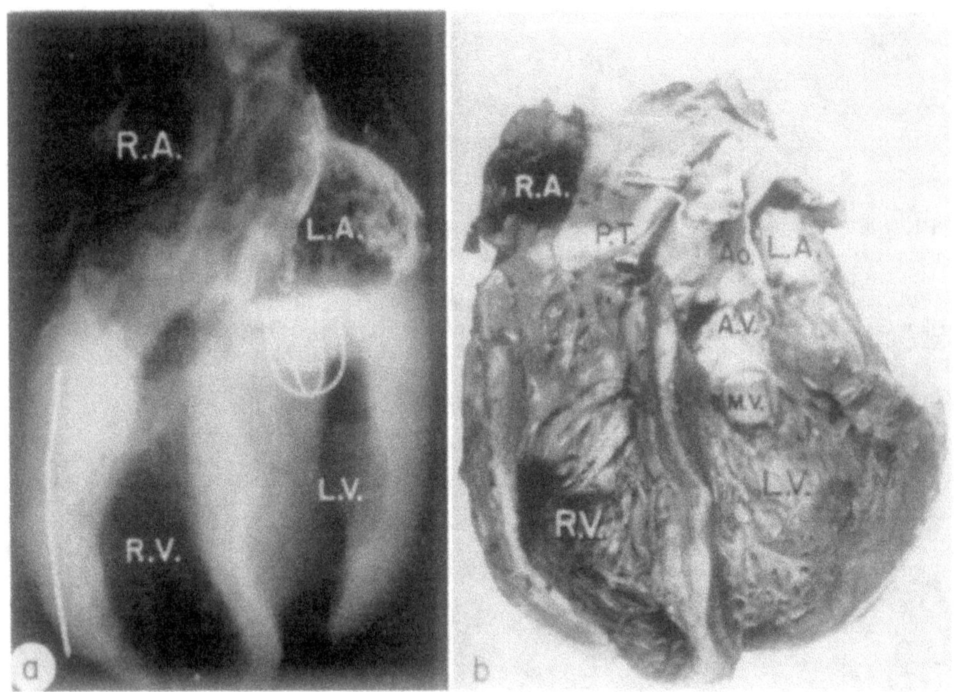

Fig. 6. Heart of Patient No. 3. a, Radiograph of excised heart, showing large calcific deposits in the left atrial (*L.A.*) wall. The mitral valve has been replaced with a Starr-Edwards prosthesis. *R.A.*, Right atrium; *R.V.*, right ventricle; *L.V.*, left ventricle. b, Opened right ventricle, pulmonary trunk (*P.T.*), left ventricle (*L.V.*), aortic valve (*A.V.*), and aorta (*Ao.*). Both ventricles are greatly enlarged. *M.V.*, Mitral valve prosthesis.

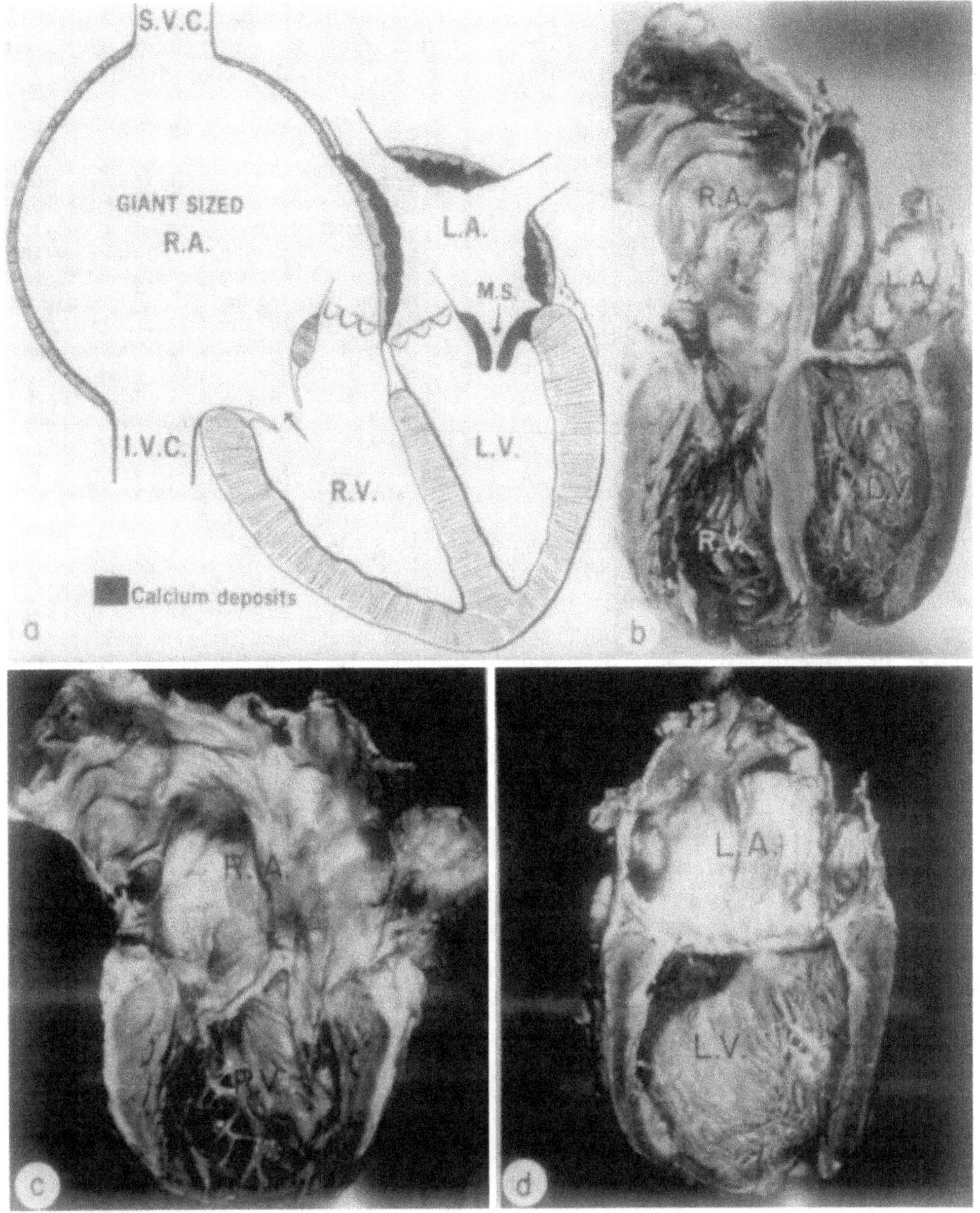

Fig. 7. Heart of Patient No. 3. *a*, Diagram. *S.V.C.*, Superior vena cava; *I.V.C.*, inferior vena cava; *R.A.*, right atrium; *R.V.*, right ventricle; *L.A.*, left atrium; *M.S.*, mitral stenosis; and *L.V.*, left ventricle. *b*, Longitudinal section of heart again showing the calcified left atrial wall and the huge right atrium. *c* and *d* are taken at the same magnification. *c*, Opened right atrium and right ventricle and *d* opened left atrium and left ventricle. The mitral prosthesis has been removed.

currence of a giant-sized right atrium with only a slightly dilated left atrium has not been specifically described. Taussig[12] noted enormous (capacity 2,150 ml.) dilatation of the right atrium and a normal-sized (capacity 100 ml.) left atrium in a 43-year-old woman with mitral and tricuspid stenosis and regurgitation, probably of rheumatic etiology, although the patient may have had the Marfan syndrome. The left atrial wall was free of calcific deposits and the heart weighed 505 grams. The cause of this unusual type of atrial dilatation is unknown.

In each of the 3 present patients the left atrial wall was calcified, the left atrium was only mildly dilated, but the right atrial cavity was huge. The hemodynamic and anatomic findings suggest that the calcium deposits in the left atrial wall prevented this chamber from dilating, decreased its compliance, and caused the elevated left atrial pressure to be immediately reflected to the pulmonary vessels and right ventricle, leading to tricuspid regurgitation of progressive severity. It seems likely that the calcification of the left atrium was the result of organization of thrombi, and in two of the patients thrombi were found at the initial operation. Each of the three patients had severe, nearly pure, mitral stenosis. Had significant or pure mitral regurgitation been present it appears unlikely that left atrial thrombi would have formed, since significantly sized left atrial thrombi have not been found, in our experience, in patients with severe mitral regurgitation.

Summary

Attention is called to the occurrence of a giant-sized right atrium and a nearly normal-sized left atrium in 3 adult patients with rheumatic mitral stenosis. In each patient the left atrial wall was calcified, probably the result of organization of intra-atrial thrombus, and the calcific deposits prevented the left atrium from dilating. All patients also had tricuspid regurgitation, which certainly contributed to the development of enormous right atrial dilatation, although other undetermined factors were probably operative also.

REFERENCES

1. Rogers, W. R., and Wittels, B.: Extreme bilateral atriomegaly. Review of the literature and report of a case, Circulation 15:434, 1957.
2. Liu, C. K., Piccirillo, R. T., and Ellestad, M.: Distensibility of the postmortem human left atrium in nonrheumatic and rheumatic heart disease, Am. J. Cardiol. 13:232, 1964.
3. Daley, R., and Franks, R.: Massive dilatation of the left atrium, Quart. J. Med. 18:81, 1949.
4. Kent, E. M., Fisher, D. L., Ford, W. B., and Neville, J. F., Jr.: Mitral valve surgery and left heart catheterization in giant left atrium, Arch. Surg. 73:503, 1956.
5. Parmley, L. F.: Congenital atriomegaly, Circulation 25:553, 1962.
6. DeSanctis, R. W., Dean, D. C., and Bland, E. F.: Extreme left atrial enlargement. Some characteristic features, Circulation 29:14, 1964.
7. Best, P. V., and Heath, D.: The right ventricle and small pulmonary arteries in aneurysmal dilatation of the left atrium, Brit. Heart J. 26:312, 1964.
8. Bishop, L. F., and Howard, E. J.: Massive left atriomegaly, Dis. Chest. 49:179, 1966.
9. Gross, L.: Lesions of the left auricle in rheumatic fever, Am. J. Path. 11:711, 1935.
10. Braunwald, E. B., and Awe, W. C.: The syndrome of severe mitral regurgitation with normal left atrial pressure, Circulation 27:29, 1963.
11. Roberts, W. C., Braunwald, E., and Morrow, A. G.: Acute severe mitral regurgitation secondary to ruptured chordae tendineae. Clinical, hemodynamic, and pathologic considerations, Circulation 33:58, 1966.
12. Taussig, B. L.: A case of tricuspid stenosis with enormous dilatation of the right auricle, Am. Heart J. 14:744, 1937.

"Mitral Stenosis" Secondary to Combined "Massive" Mitral Anular Calcific Deposits and Small, Hypertrophied Left Ventricles

Hemodynamic Documentation in Four Patients

WILLIAM J. HAMMER, M.D.

Philadelphia, Pennsylvania

WILLIAM C. ROBERTS, M.D.

Bethesda, Maryland

ANTONIO C. deLEON, Jr., M.D.

Washington, D. C.

From the Division of Cardiology, Department of Medicine, Georgetown University Medical Center, Washington, D.C.; and the Pathology Branch, National Heart, Lung and Blood Institute, National Institutes of Health, Bethesda, Maryland. This study was supported in part by the Benjamin May Memorial Fund. Requests for reprints should be addressed to Dr. Antonio C. deLeon, Jr., Division of Cardiology, Department of Medicine, Georgetown University Medical Center, 3800 Reservoir Road, N.W., Washington, D.C. 20007. Manuscript accepted June 22, 1977.

Certain observations are described in four elderly women with massive mitral anular calcific deposits, small thick-walled left ventricles and diastolic gradients between pulmonary artery wedge position (or left atrium) and left ventricle. All four patients had some degree of obstruction to left ventricular outflow. Examination at necropsy (two patients) or at operation (one patient) disclosed only focal fibrous thickening of the mitral leaflets without commissural or chordal fusion. By auscultation, none had mitral opening snaps, only two had loud first heart sounds and only one had a mitral diastolic rumble. Hemodynamic documentation of a diastolic gradient between pulmonary artery wedge position (or left atrium) and left ventricle in the presence of massive mitral anular calcific deposits and in the absence of diffuse disease of the mitral leaflets has not been demonstrated previously. The diastolic gradients are considered to result from the combination of the large mitral anular calcific deposits and the small, thick-walled, noncompliant left ventricles.

Although calcific deposits in the mitral anulus are extremely common [1], mainly in older persons, the hemodynamic consequences of these deposits are poorly understood. When the deposits are relatively small, i.e., not visible roentgenologically, it is unlikely that valvular dysfunction results. Large deposits, i.e., those visible during life by roentgenogram, of anular calcium, however, may be associated with mild to moderate degrees of mitral regurgitation but probably never severe regurgitation [1,2]. Although apical diastolic murmurs have been observed and stenosis of this valve suspected at necropsy in some patients with "massive" mitral anular calcific deposits [3], hemodynamic documentation of diastolic gradients between pulmonary artery wedge position (or left atrium) and left ventricle in patients with "massive" calcific deposits of the mitral anulus has not been reported. The present communication describes observations in four such patients.

PATIENTS STUDIED AND METHODS

Certain clinical and hemodynamic observations in the four patients are presented in Table I. Three patients had angina pectoris and two had syncope. None had a history of acute rheumatic fever. The mean pressure gradients

TABLE I   Clinical and Hemodynamic Observations in the Four Patients Studied with Massive Calcific Deposits in the Mitral Anulus and Small Hypertrophied Left Ventricles

Case No.	Age (yrs) and Sex	Rhythm	S_1	OS	S_3	S_4	Murmur (grade 0–6) of					Hemodynamics (mm Hg)							Angiogram		
							MS	MR	AS	AR	HC	PA (s/d)	PAW a	PAW v	PAW m	LV (s/d)	SA s/d	PAW-LV mdg	LV-SA psg	MR (0–4)	AR (0–4)
1	70,F	Sinus ↑	0	+	+	0	2	5	0	0	46/22	34	46	30	268/4	115/60	15	153	1	1
2	70,F	Sinus ↑	0	+	+	1	0	2	2	0	45/22	33	28	22	179/22	170/90	15	9	1	1
3	74,F	Sinus N	0	0	+	0	0	3	1	0	26/6	14*	6*	6*	210/5	120/80	8*	90	—	—
4	70,F	AF	Va	+	0	0	2	0	0	2	100/55	—	60	35	160/20†	95/60	21	65†	4	0

NOTE: A = a wave; AF = atrial fibrillation; AR = aortic regurgitation; AS = aortic stenosis; HC = hypertrophic cardiomyopathy; LV = left ventricle; m = mean; mdg = mean diastolic gradient; MR = mitral regurgitation; MS = mitral stenosis; N = normal; OS = opening snap; PAW = pulmonary arterial wedge; psg = peak systolic gradient; SA = systemic artery; S_1 = first heart sound; S_3 = ventricular diastolic gallop; S_4 = atrial diastolic gallop; s/d = peak systole/end diastole; v = v wave; Va = variable.

* Left atrial rather than pulmonary artery wedge pressure.

† On pullback from left ventricle to aorta the peak systolic pressure gradient was 120 mm Hg (LV body, 200/20; LV outflow, 80/20; aorta, 80/60 mm Hg).

between pulmonary arterial wedge position (left atrium in one patient) and left ventricle in the four patients ranged from 8 to 21 mm Hg (average 14.7 mm Hg) (Figures 1 and 2). In addition to these pressure gradients, all four patients also had left ventricular outflow tract obstruction: from valvular stenosis in three and from hypertrophic cardiomyopathy in one.

By auscultation, only one patient had an apical diastolic rumble, two had apical holosystolic murmurs consistent with mitral regurgitation, four had murmurs of aortic stenosis, and two of aortic regurgitation. By angiography, however, three had evidence of mitral regurgitation and two of aortic regurgitation. Of the three patients with sinus rhythm, the first heart sound was increased in intensity in one. Fourth hearth sounds were present in three patients, and third heart sounds in three patients. None had mitral opening snaps. All four had mitral anular calcific deposits large enough to be visible by routine chest roentgenogram; three also had calcific deposits in the aortic valve (Figure 3). The electrocardiogram showed normal sinus rhythm in three, atrial fibrillation in one, left ventricular hypertrophy in three, left atrial abnormality in two and right ventricular hypertrophy in none. Echocardiograms in two patients (Cases 1 and 2) disclosed large echoes in the region behind the posterior mitral leaflet. The E-F slope of the an-

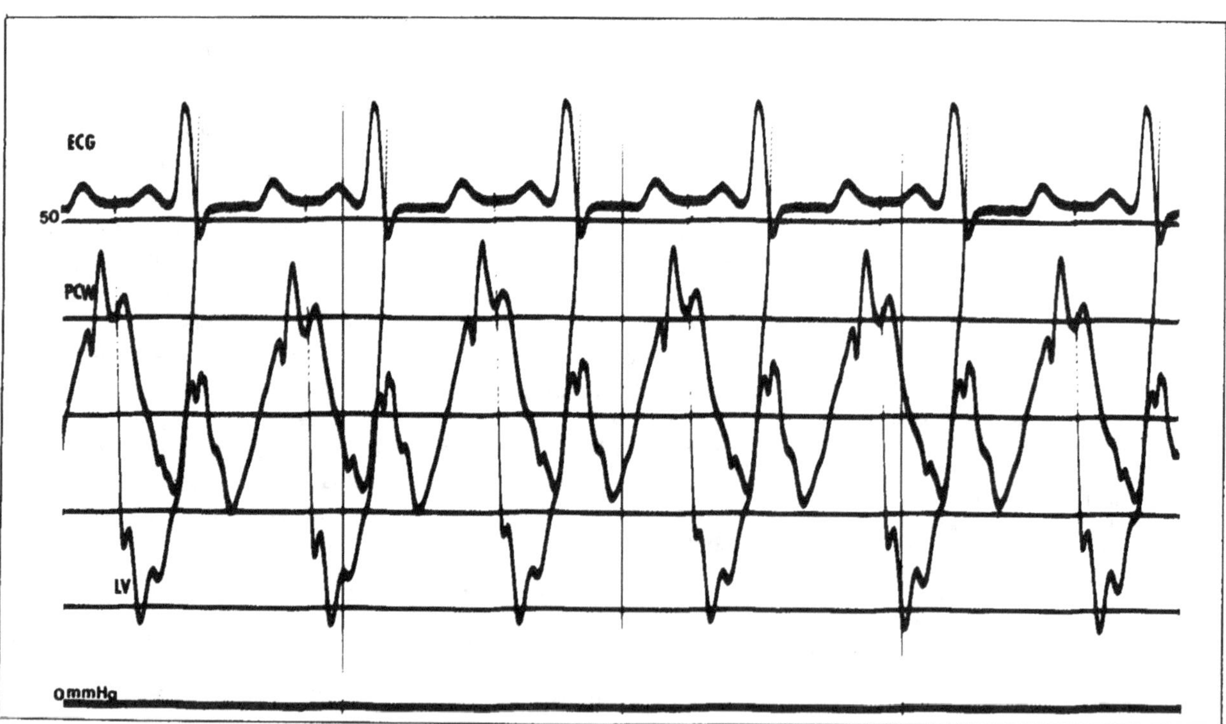

Figure 1. Simultaneous, equisensitive recording of pulmonary arterial wedge (PCW) and left ventricular pressures (LV) in patient (Case 2) demonstrating a sizable diastolic gradient.

terior mitral leaflet could not be satisfactorily demonstrated because of the large echoes from massive anular calcification.

Each of the two patients with significant valvular aortic stenosis underwent aortic valve replacement. The aortic valve was congenitally bicuspid in one (Case 1) (Figure 3) and three-cuspid without commissural fusion, the type most commonly seen in the elderly [1], in the other. The anterior mitral leaflet in both were freely mobile. One of these two patients died early, and necropsy confirmed the presence of massive mitral anular calcific deposits (Figure 3) and, other than focal aging changes, an otherwise normal mitral valve. Another patient (Case 3) died late after aortic valve replacement and necropsy was not performed. The third patient (Case 2) did not have surgery and is living. In none of the patients was a procedure performed on the mitral valve. One patient (Case 4) had hypertrophic cardiopathy and died of congestive cardiac failure. At necropsy, the mitral leaflets and chordae tendineae were quite mobile but focally thickened, and the amount of anular calcific deposits was large. In neither of the two necropsy patients was the chordae or commissures fused or the leaflets more than just focally thickened; in both, the calcific deposits were limited to the area behind the posterior mitral leaflets. In three patients, the left ventricular cavity appeared smaller than normal by left ventricular angiography (two patients) or by necropsy examination (two patients). The left ventricular cavity was judged "normal" by angiography in one patient (Case 2).

COMMENTS

Each of the four patients described in this report was a woman aged 70 years or older, each had "massive" deposits of calcium in the mitral anular region, each had diastolic gradients between pulmonary artery wedge position (of left atrium) and left ventricle, each had a relatively small left ventricular cavity and a hypertrophied left ventricular wall, and each had obstruction to left ventricular outflow. Other than focal fibrous thickening of the leaflets (the result of aging or hypertrophic cardiomyopathy, or both) disease of the mitral leaflets or chordae clearly was not the cause of the diastolic gradient. It is likely that the small and thick-walled left ventricles in association with the large mitral anular calcific deposits were responsible for the diastolic gradients. The small areas available for left ventricular inflow because of the left ventricular hypertrophy without dilatation were further compromised by the huge deposits of calcium behind the posterior mitral leaflets. That the small, thick-walled left ventricles did contribute to the diastolic gradients is supported by the lack of diastolic gradients in other patients with similarly large mitral anular calcific deposits and large left ventricular cavities (Figure 4). Although it is recognized that severe mitral regurgitation may further augment the degree of mitral stenosis, only one of the four patients (Case 4) had substantial mitral regurgitation by left ventricular angiography, one had none, and in two it was trivial. The unusually tall V waves and angiographically demonstrated 4+ mitral regurgitation in one patient (Case 4) indicated severe mitral regurgitation. The increased level of mean left atrial pressure caused by the mitral regurgitation may be a factor in the large (21 mm Hg)

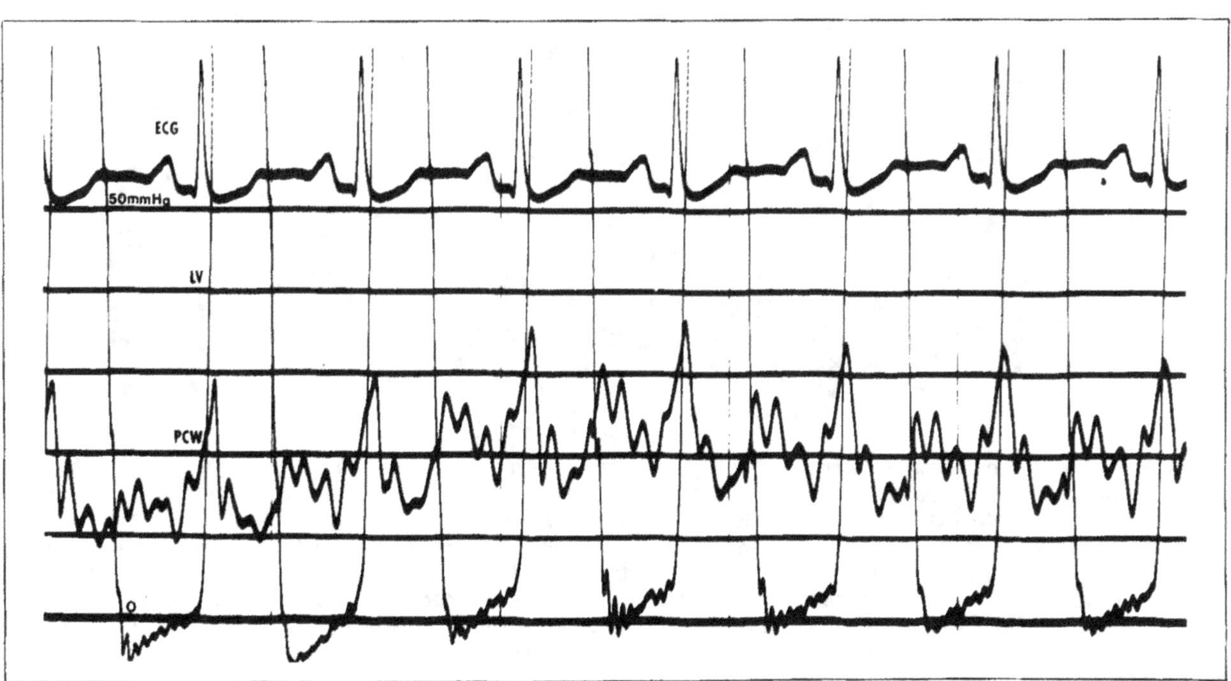

Figure 2. Simultaneous, equisensitive recording of pulmonary arterial wedge (PCW) and left ventricular pressures (LV) in patient (Case 1) demonstrating a diastolic gradient.

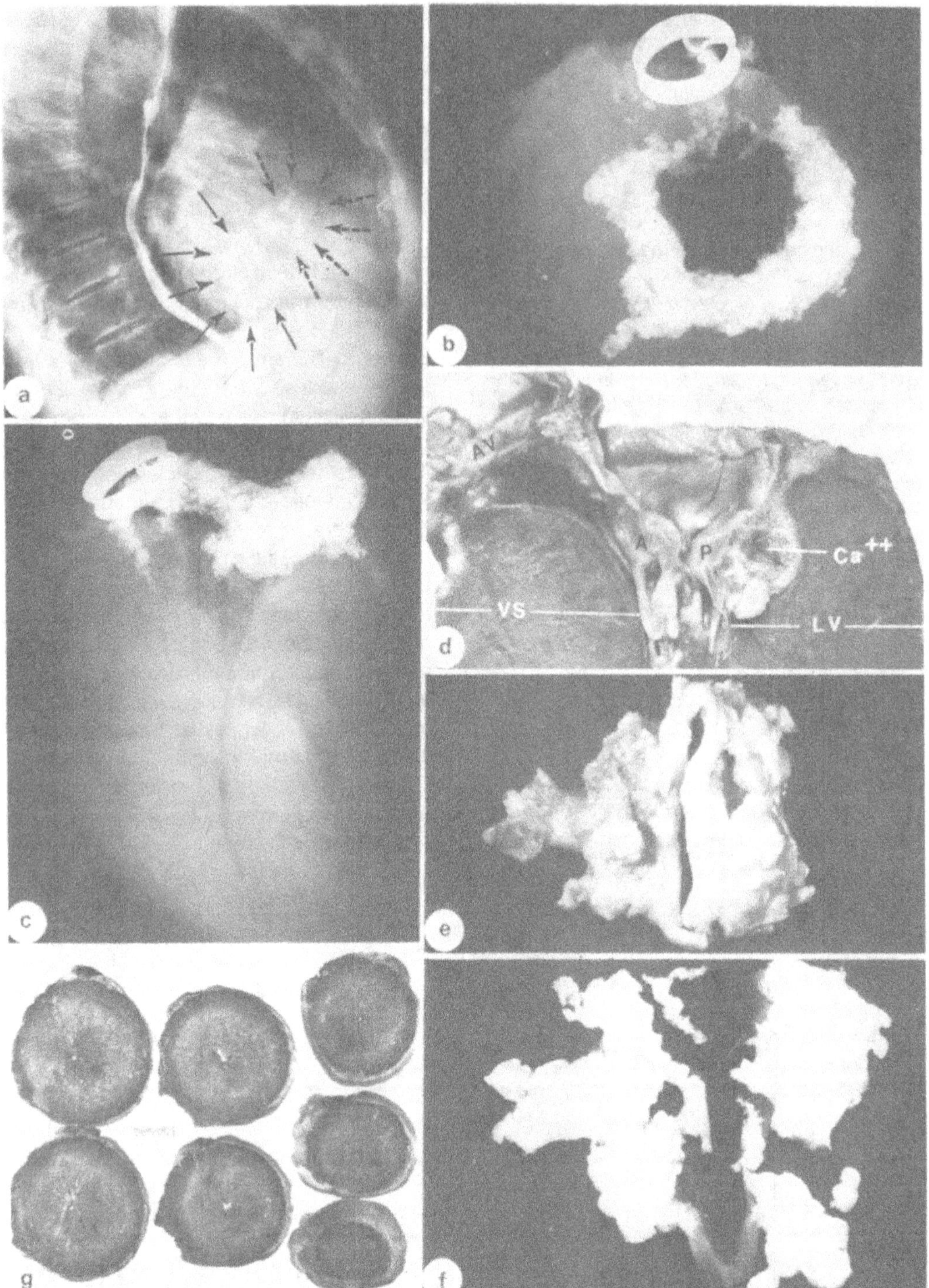

Figure 3. Case 1. Chest roentgenogram (**a**), roentgenograms of the heart specimen (**b,c,f**) and photographs of the heart (**d,e,g**) in patient (Case 1). **a**, a u-shaped deposit of calcium in the mitral anular region (solid arrows) and another deposit of calcium in the aortic valve (dashed arrows) are apparent in this lateral view. **b**, this postmortem film shows the extent of the mitral anular calcific deposit. The aortic valve has been replaced by a Bjork-Shiley prosthesis. **c**, lateral view of the heart. The left ventricular cavity is minute. **d**, basal portion of left ventricle (LV) showing the anterior (A) and posterior (P) mitral leaflets and aortic valve (AV) area from which the tilting disc prosthesis was excised at necropsy. A large deposit of calcium is present behind, and attached to, the posterior mitral leaflet. VS = ventricular septum. **e**, operatively excised stenotic, bicuspid aortic valve. **f**, film of the excised aortic valve. **g**, transverse sections of the left ventricle (the right ventricular free wall was excised from these slices) showing a minute left ventricular cavity.

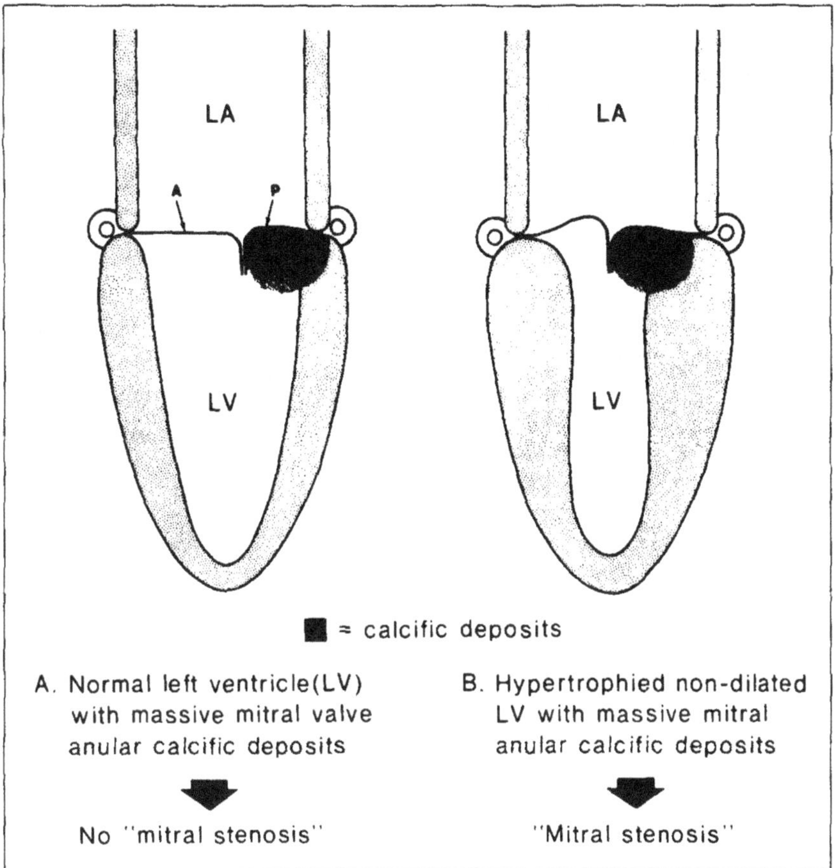

Figure 4. *Diagram showing the probable mechanism of the diastolic gradients in our patients. In both diagrams, the size of the mitral anular calcific deposits is similar and quite large. In **A** the left ventricular wall and cavity are normal. In **B** the left ventricular wall is considerably hypertrophied and the cavity is smaller than normal. The combination of the large calcific deposits in the mitral anulus in association with a small, thick-walled left ventricle is sufficient to produce a diastolic gradient whereas none results when the left ventricular cavity is enlarged and its wall thickness, normal.*

mean diastolic gradient in this case. However, it is unlikely that mitral regurgitation contributed in any significant degree to the mitral diastolic gradient in three of our four patients. The significant degree of pulmonary hypertension in this patient is in part due to the increased left atrial pressure, but abnormal pulmonary vascular resistance must also be a contributing factor. Pathologically, medial hypertrophy and intimal proliferation causing luminal narrowing of the smaller pulmonary arteries were present. The etiology of this could not be definitively determined.

The auscultatory findings in our four patients differed from the classic findings of rheumatic mitral stenosis [4]. Only two of the four patients had a loud first heart sound (S_1), none had a mitral opening snap, and only one had an apical diastolic rumble. The left ventricular outflow obstruction with resulting increase in left ventricular pressure, left ventricular hypertrophy and increased rate of left ventricular pressure (dp/dt), might

explain the loud first heart sound in our two patients. The focal rather than diffuse nature of the mitral leaflet thickening may explain the absence of an opening snap in our patients. The consistent presence of rapid filling sounds (S4 and/or S3) presents an additional paradox in view of the mitral gradients. The presence of the diastolic filling sounds imply rapid blood flow into the left ventricle. One could postulate, therefore, that the degree of mitral valve obstruction was mild. Yet, in three of our patients, the measured mean resting mitral valve gradient was 15 and 21 mm Hg, suggesting severe obstruction. The mitral valves of the two patients examined at necropsy provide evidence that central rapid flow between the left atrium and left ventricle is possible. The additional presence of a small left ventricular cavity with stiff, relatively noncompliant left ventricular walls may explain the genesis of the diastolic filling sounds. It is certainly possible that the small left ventricular cavity in diastole and/or markedly diminished compliance of the left ventricular wall somehow plays a role in the genesis of the mitral diastolic pressure gradient. Rapid flow from the left atrium to the left ventricle is possible, but the volume of flow may be limited by the relatively small left ventricular cavity, resulting in lack of diastasis during the available diastolic filling period. This proposed mechanism can explain the paradox of rapid filling sound (S4 and/or S3) and presence of substantial pressure gradient across the mitral valve. Thus, because of a different mechanism for obstruction, its clinical presentation is different from that seen in rheumatic mitral stenosis. Massive mitral anular calcification represents a heretofore unemphasized cause of "obstruction" at the mitral valve level.

REFERENCES

1. Roberts WC, Perloff JK: Mitral valvular disease. A clinicopathologic survey of the conditions causing the mitral valve to function abnormally. Ann Intern Med 77: 939, 1972.
2. Perloff K, Roberts WC: The mitral apparatus. Functional anatomy of mitral regurgitation. Circulation 46: 227, 1972.
3. Korn D, DeSanctis RW, Sell S: Massive calcification of the mitral anulus. A clinicopathological study of fourteen cases. N Engl J Med 267: 900, 1962.
4. Reichek N, Shelburne JC, Perloff JK: Clinical aspects of rheumatic valvular disease. Prog Cardiovasc Dis 15: 491, 1973.

Aschoff Bodies *At Necropsy* in Valvular Heart Disease

Evidence from an Analysis of 543 Patients Over 14 Years of Age that Rheumatic Heart Disease, At Least Anatomically, Is a Disease of the Mitral Valve

WILLIAM C. ROBERTS, M.D., AND RENU VIRMANI, M.D.

SUMMARY Among 543 necropsy patients over age 14 years with severe chronic valvular heart disease, Aschoff bodies were found in 11 patients (2%). The ages of the 11 patients ranged from 18 to 68 years (avg 38), and nine had had a history of acute rheumatic fever earlier in life. Clinically, nine of the 11 patients had mitral stenosis with or without dysfunction of one or more other cardiac valves, one had isolated aortic regurgitation, and one had both mitral and aortic regurgitation. All 11 patients had diffuse fibrous thickening of the mitral valve leaflets, and all but one had diffuse anatomic lesions of at least one other cardiac valve. No patient with anatomic lesions limited to the aortic valve had Aschoff bodies. Thus, among patients with chronic valvular heart disease, Aschoff bodies, the only anatomic lesion pathognomonic of rheumatic heart disease, indicate diffuse anatomic lesions of the mitral leaflets and usually also anatomic lesions of one or more other cardiac valves. The functional mitral lesion is usually stenosis.

SINCE ASCHOFF[1] first described in 1904 lesions in the heart which have subsequently become known as *Aschoff bodies,* these lesions have been sought at necropsy in patients with valvular heart disease. Of 518 necropsy patients with valvular heart disease reported from 1934 to 1961 (table 1), the percent with Aschoff bodies varied enormously (from 9 to 84% [avg 42]).[2-12] These 11 previous studies (table 1)[2-12] were based on variable and often unclear criteria for defining Aschoff bodies. Because of this marked variation in reported frequency of Aschoff bodies in necropsy patients and because of a previous study by us on the frequency of Aschoff bodies in operatively excised atrial appendage and papillary muscle,[13] it appeared worthwhile to examine a large number of necropsy patients with chronic valvular heart disease to determine the frequency and clinical significance of Aschoff bodies.

Patients Studied and Methods

All patients with chronic valvular heart disease in whom necropsy was performed at the Clinical Center of the National Institutues of Health and all necropsy patients with valvular heart disease in whom the heart was submitted to the Pathology Branch of the National Heart, Lung, and Blood Institute between 1953 and 1972 were included in this analysis. A total of 543 necropsy patients with severe (functional class III or IV, New York Heart Association classification) chronic valvular heart disease was analyzed (table 2). Each of the 543 hearts was examined grossly and histologically by one of us (WCR) and the cases were classified according to the functional valve lesion detected clinically (table 2). Tricuspid regurgitation, however, was not included in the functional classification. In over 90% of the 543 patients, the functional valve lesions had been confirmed by, or diagnosed by, cardiac catheterization with or without angiography. In addition to classifying the patients by their functional valve lesions, each was also classified anatomically. Some patients with clinically isolated mitral stenosis, for example, at necropsy also had diffuse anatomic lesions of the aortic valve. Therefore, these patients were classified anatomically as mitral plus aortic but clinically only as mitral stenosis (table 2). Also, for a valve to be considered abnormal anatomically there must have been *diffuse* thickening of all portions of each valve cusp or thickening of the *margins* around the entire valve circumference (fig. 1). Focal leaflet thickening, i.e., sparing at least some marginal areas, was not considered indicative of anatomic abnormality.

Of the 543 patients, their ages at death ranged from 15 to 88 years (avg 45); 64% were men and 36%, women. A cardiac operation (valve commissurotomy, anuloplasty or replacement) had been performed in 372 (69%) of the 543 patients.

At least one section of wall of each cardiac chamber was cut, processed, stained (hematoxylin-eosin) and examined histologically. Each section included the through-and-through thickness of wall from endocardium to epicardium. Each section for histologic study was at least 2 cm in maximal dimension. At least four histologic sections were examined from each patient, an average of seven per patient. The criteria used for recognizing Aschoff bodies are those proposed by Saphir[14] and summarized in table 3.

Results

Aschoff bodies were found in the heart in 11 (2%) of the 543 patients (table 2). The frequency of the Aschoff bodies in these 11 patients were *numerous* in six, *many* in one, and *rare* in four. The patients with either numerous or many Aschoff bodies had these structures in the walls of at least three of the four cardiac chambers and multiple ones were observed in the sections. In contrast, the patients with rare Aschoff bodies had these structures in the walls of only one or two chambers: in two patients, only in left ventricle, and in the other two, both left ventricle and left atrium. In the four patients with rare Aschoff bodies, only three to six of these structures were observed per patient in all the sections

From the Pathology Branch, National Heart, Lung, and Blood Institute, National Institutes of Health, Bethesda, Maryland.

Address for reprints: William C. Roberts, M.D., Building 10A, Room 3E-30, National Institutes of Health, Bethesda, Maryland 20014.

Received May 30, 1977; revision accepted November 22, 1977.

TABLE 1. *Reported Frequency of Aschoff Bodies At Necropsy in Valvular Heart Disease*

First author	Year (Ref. No.)	No. of patients	No. (%) with Aschoff Bodies	No. (%) pts. with MS
Rothschild	1934 (2)	161	95 (59)	—
McKeown	1945 (3)	18	15 (84)	12 (67)
Pinniger	1951 (4)	19	6 (31)	19 (100)
Waaler	1952 (5)	16	5 (31)	16 (100)
McKeown	1953 (6)	92	22 (25)	92 (100)
Decker	1953 (7)	22	6 (27)	22 (100)
Thomas	1953 (8)	40	29 (72)	40 (100)
Luse	1954 (9)	28	3 (11)	28 (100)
Tedeschi	1955 (10)	22	2 (9)	22 (100)
Lannigan	1959 (11)	76	27 (35)	76 (100)
Ruebner	1961 (12)	24	8 (33)	24 (100)
Totals		518	218 (42)	343/358 (96)

MS = mitral stenosis.

examined. In two patients, Aschoff bodies also were observed in epicardium and each of these patients had numerous Aschoff bodies. In all 11 patients Aschoff bodies were observed in both mural endocardium and in myocardium. Aschoff bodies were not observed in valvular endocardium in any patient but sections of valve were not examined in all patients. The number of histologic sections of heart examined in each of the 11 patients with Aschoff bodies ranged from 6 to 16 (avg 10).

The *functional* and *anatomic* valvular lesions in the 11 patients with Aschoff bodies are summarized in table 4. Of the 11 patients, nine had mitral stenosis with or without functional lesions of other cardiac valves, one had pure aortic regurgitation and one had both aortic and mitral regurgitation. Although only 18 functional valve lesions (excluding tricuspid regurgitation) were observed in the 11 patients with Aschoff bodies, 26 anatomic valve lesions were present in these patients. All 11 patients had anatomic lesions of the mitral valve (fig. 1), ten had anatomic involvement of the aortic valve, four also of the tricuspid valve, and one also of the pulmonic valve. Thus, of the 11 patients, only one had anatomic lesions limited to only one valve (mitral), and the other ten had anatomic lesions of two or more valves.

Certain clinical features in the 11 necropsy patients with Aschoff bodies are summarized in table 5 and these observations are compared to those in our previous study[14] of 45 surgical patients with Aschoff bodies in operatively excised atrial appendage or papillary muscle.

Comments

The last reported study describing the frequency of Aschoff bodies *at necropsy* in patients with valvular heart disease appeared in 1961 and concerned only 24 patients.[12] The largest previous study on this subject appeared in 1934 and concerned 161 patients.[2] Although several studies on the frequency of Aschoff bodies at necropsy appeared between 1934 and 1961, none provided much clinical information regarding the patients with Aschoff bodies, few described the relative frequency of distribution of the Aschoff bodies in the heart, and none described the number(s) of cardiac valves involved anatomically or functionally other than mitral

TABLE 2. *Functional Classification of Valvular Heart Disease. Data in 543 Necropsy Patients > Age 14 Years*

Functional valve lesion	Patients No. (%)	Age range in years (Avg)	Non-rheumatic etiology No. (%)	Rheumatic etiology No. (%)	Rheumatics with hx ARF or Chorea No. (%)	Total with hx ARF or Chorea No. (%)	Anatomic valve lesion(s): No. (%)					No. (%) with Aschoff bodies
							AV	MV	MV + AV	MV + TV	MV + AV + TV	
Aortic stenosis (AS)	182 (34)	16-90 (48)	159 (87)	23 (13)	14 (61)	22 (12)	158 (87)	0	23 (12.5)	0	1 (.5)	0
Mitral stenosis (MS)	94 (17)	21-85 (46)	0	94 (100)	61 (65)	61 (65)	0	53 (57)	23 (24)	7 (7)	11 (12)	3 (3)
AS + MS	66 (12)	28-81 (50)	0	66 (100)	51 (77)	51 (77)	0	0	52 (79)	0	14 (21)	5 (8)
Aortic regurgitation (AR)	60 (11)	15-69 (41)	50 (83)	10 (17)	9 (90)	12 (20)	50 (83)	0	9 (15)	0	1 (2)	1 (2)
Mitral regurgitation (MR)	55 (10)	15-78 (40)	25 (45)	30 (55)	20 (67)	20 (36)	0	44 (80)	7 (13)	1 (2)	3 (5)	0
MS + AR	34 (6)	23-71 (44)	0	34 (100)	27 (80)	27 (80)	0	0	25 (74)	0	9 (26)	1 (3)
MR + AR	24 (5)	20-65 (38)	5 (21)	19 (79)	17 (71)	17 (71)	0	0	20 (83)	0	4 (17)	1 (4)
MR + AS	16 (3)	25-80 (51)	0	16 (100)	11 (69)	11 (69)	0	0	15 (94)	0	1 (6)	0
Tricuspid stenosis + MS ± AS	12 (2)	31-52 (39)	0	12 (100)	9 (75)	9 (75)	0	0	0	1 (8)	11 (92)	0
Totals	543	15-90 (45)	240 (44)	303 (56)	219 (72)	231 (43)	208 (38)	97 (18)	174 (32)	9 (2)	55 (10)	11 (2)

Abbreviations: ARF = acute rheumatic fever; AV = aortic valve; Hx = history of; MV = mitral valve; TV = tricuspid valve.

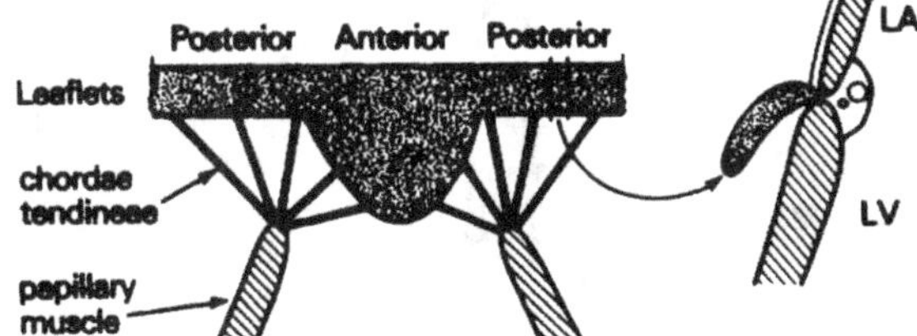

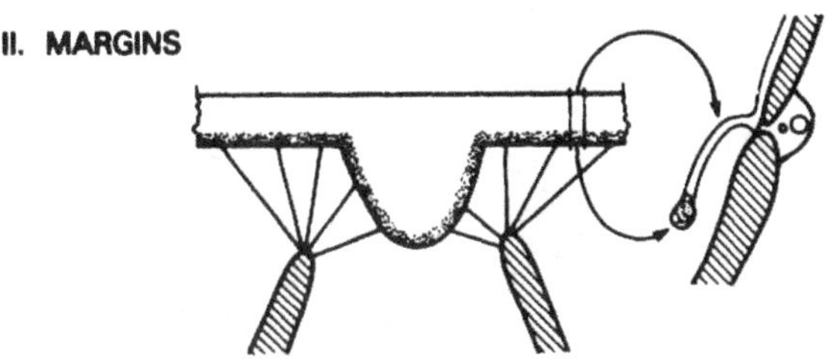

▨ Portion of Leaflets Abnormal Structurally

FIGURE 1. *Diagram showing the two types of anatomic involvement of the mitral valve in rheumatic heart disease.*

TABLE 3. *The Aschoff Nodule: Histologic Features*

1. Round or oval shape
2. Located only in endocardium or perivascular regions.
3. Consists of a variety of cells arranged more or less in several parallel rows.
   A. *Cardiac histocyte* (also called Antischkow cell or myocyte, Aschoff cell, and myocardial reticulocyte)—its cytoplasm is slightly basophilic (on hematoxylin-eosin stain) and its nucleus is clearly outlined, vesicular and oval. Its chromatin is arranged in bars and appears spiderlike. The area around the chromatin is clear. On cross section, the chromatin appears as a dark spot surrounded by clear area. These cells may have 2 or 3 centrally placed and overlapping nuclei.
   B. *Lymphocytes*—few
   C. *Polymorphonuclear leukocytes*—occasional
   D. *Mast cell*—rare
4. Foci of fibrinoid degeneration or necrosis or both are present between and adjacent to the cells.

[Modified from Saphir O: The Aschoff nodule. Am J Clin Pathol 31:534, 1959].

stenosis. In the present study a larger group of patients, 543, were examined than in all the previous studies combined. Furthermore, the types of functional and anatomic valvular lesions in our 543 patients were classified by reexamination of all 543 hearts by the same examiner and a relatively large number of histologic sections were examined from each heart. Despite this extensive search, the frequency of Aschoff bodies in our patients who died between 1953 and 1971 was surprisingly low, only 2%. The large difference in the low frequency (11 of 543) of Aschoff bodies in our patients with chronic valvular heart disease compared to the high frequency (218 [42%] of 518) in the reported patients dying between the 1920s and 1961 (table 1)[2-12] is uncertain. Presumably, differences in histologic criteria used to diagnose Aschoff bodies explains some of the difference. Also, the more frequent use of penicillin in our patients also may have prevented repeated attacks of acute rheumatic fever.[15] Although the ages of the reported necropsy patients were available in only two previous studies,[6,12] it is likely that our patients were on the average older than those described in the previous reports (table 1). Our study, for example, excluded patients under 15 years of age. The composition of our 543 patients, most of whom were studied at one institution, probably differed considerably from that of the previously reported 518 patients from multiple institutions. Almost surely the frequency of isolated aortic stenosis was greater in our study patients (182 of the 543) and none of them had Aschoff bodies at necropsy. Aschoff bodies, to our knowledge, have never been described in a patient with isolated aortic valve lesions. In contrast, of the 357 previously reported patients in whom the functional valve lesion was mentioned, 343 (96%) had mitral stenosis. Among our 543 patients, 206 had mitral stenosis, with or without a functional lesion involving other cardiac valves, and only 9 (4%) of them had Aschoff bodies. Thus, it is likely that the incidence of Aschoff bodies is dropping in patients with chronic valvular heart disease just as is the incidence of acute rheumatic fever itself.[15]

Although the presence of Aschoff bodies nearly always indicates the presence of mitral stenosis (table 1), there are exceptions. Of our 11 patients with Aschoff bodies, nine had mitral stenosis but the other two had purely regurgitant lesions — purely aortic in one, and combined aortic and mitral in the other. Although mitral stenosis is not quite uni-

TABLE 4. *Aschoff Bodies at Necropsy (in 543 Patients > Age 14 Years)*

Patient	Age	Sex	Hx ARF	Valve(s) Scarred	Functional Valve Lesion(s)	Frequency Aschoff Bodies	Rhythm
1	56	M	+	MV	MS	Numerous	AF
2	39	F	+	MV–AV	MS	Rare	AF
3	40	M	+	MV–AV	MS–AS	Rare	AF
4	30	F	+	MV–AV	MR–AR	Numerous	Sinus
5	47	F	+	MV–AV	MS–AS	Rare	Sinus
6	68	M	+	MV–AV	MS–AS	Numerous	Sinus
7	33	F	0	MV–AV	MS–AS	Rare	AF
8	39	F	+	MV–AV–TV	MS–AS	Numerous	AF
9	18	F	0	MV–AV–TV	MS	Numerous	AF
10	19	M	+	MV–AV–TV	AR	Numerous	Sinus
11	31	M		MV–AV–TV–PV	MS–AR	Many	AF

Abbreviations: AF = atrial fibrillation; ARF = acute rheumatic fever; AS = aortic stenosis; AR = aortic regurgitation; AV = aortic valve; Hx = history; MS = mitral stenosis; MV = mitral valve; PV = pulmonic valve, and TV = tricuspid valve.

TABLE 5. *Clinical Observations in Patients with Aschoff Bodies At Necropsy (11 Patients) or At Operation (45 Patients)**

	11 necropsy patients	45 surgical patients*
Ages at operation or necropsy	18-68 (avg 38)	10-54 Years (avg 32)
Males:Females	5:6	20:25
White:Black:Other	All white	37:3:5
Mitral stenosis	9	44
Pure mitral regurgitation	1**	1
History of ARF	9 (82%)	26 (58%)
Age at 1st ARF	9-68 (avg 25)	4-26 (avg 13)
ASO Titer normal	—	100% (26/26)
Streptococci in throat culture	—	0 (0/13)
Sinus rhythm	4 (36%)	38 (84%)
Atrial fibrillation	7 (64%)	7 (16%)
PA systolic pressure >50 mm Hg	4 (36%)	20 (43%)

*Data from reference 13.
**Patient also had pure aortic regurgitation. An additional patient had isolated pure aortic regurgitation.
Abbreviations: ARF = acute rheumatic fever; ASO = antistreptolysin O titer; PA = pulmonary artery.

versal in patients with Aschoff bodies, the presence of diffuse or marginal anatomic lesions (fig. 1) of the mitral valve does appear to be universal among the patients with Aschoff bodies. Mitral stenosis, obviously, always indicates diffuse anatomic lesions of the mitral leaflets. In each of our two patients without mitral stenosis but with Aschoff bodies, both, nevertheless, had diffuse anatomic lesions of the mitral leaflets, in one causing no mitral valve dysfunction and in the second causing pure mitral regurgitation. Among the 45 surgical patients in whom Aschoff bodies were observed by us in either atrial appendage or papillary muscle or both, 44 had mitral stenosis, and the remaining one, a 10-year-old boy, had pure mitral regurgitation.[14] Thus, all 45 had diffuse anatomic lesions of the mitral valve. Accordingly, we define rheumatic heart disease as a disease *at least anatomically* of the mitral valve (fig. 1). Other valves also may be involved either anatomically or functionally or both, but always the mitral valve is involved anatomically, either diffusely or at their margins, and, with rare exception, the functional mitral lesion is stenosis, with or without regurgitation, and rarely, pure regurgitation.

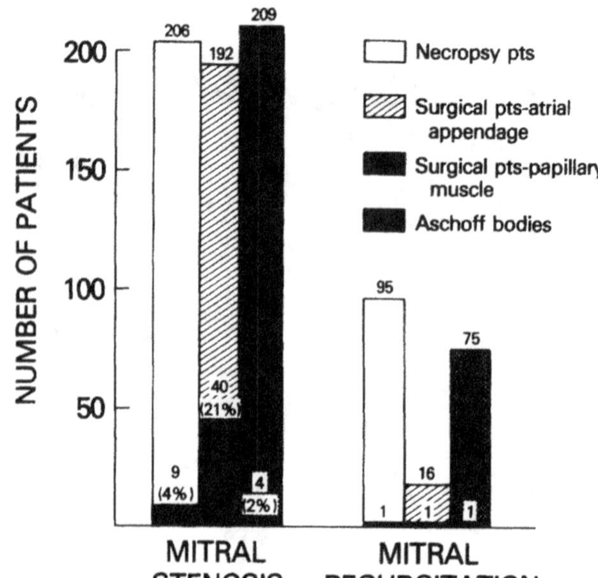

FIGURE 2. *Frequency of Aschoff bodies in necropsy and surgical patients with either mitral stenosis or pure mitral regurgitation with or without dysfunction of one or more other cardiac valves.*

The frequency of Aschoff bodies in our 543 *necropsy* patients is significantly ($P < 0.01$) different from the frequency in our 481 *surgical* patients (previously described[14]) in whom the left atrial appendage or left ventricular papillary muscle or both were examined histologically. The frequency of Aschoff bodies in the necropsy patients was 2% and in the surgical patients, 9%. This comparison, however, has deficiencies because the necropsy patients include a large number, namely 182, with disease only of the aortic valve, whereas the surgical group excludes patients with aortic valve disease. Thus, among the 301 *necropsy* patients with only mitral valve disease, either stenosis or pure mitral regurgitation or both, with or without involvement of other cardiac valves, Aschoff bodies were found in 10 (3%); in contrast, among the 481 *surgical* patients with mitral valve disease, 45 (9%) had Aschoff bodies ($P < 0.01$).

Because Aschoff bodies are observed most frequently in patients with mitral stenosis, comparison of the necropsy and surgical patients with this particular lesion is more

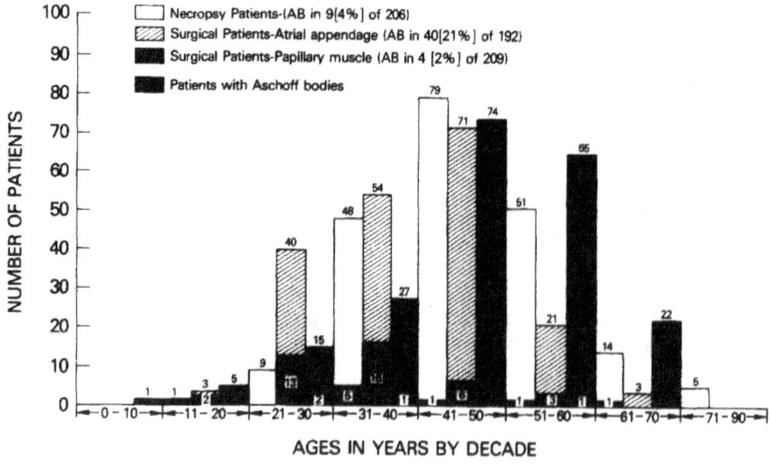

FIGURE 3. *Frequency by decade of Aschoff bodies (AB) in necropsy and surgical patients with mitral stenosis with or without dysfunction of other cardiac valves.*

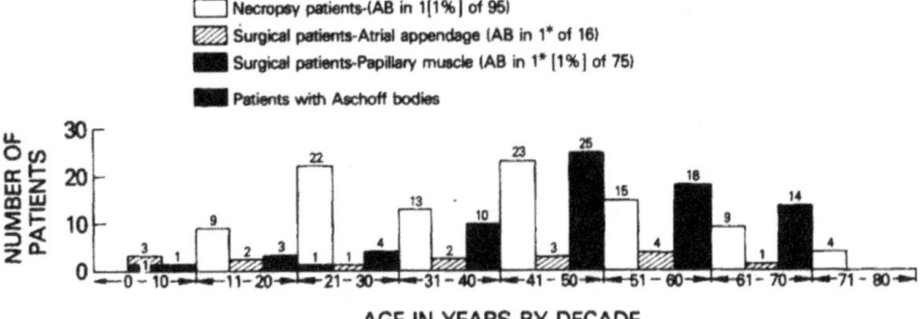

FIGURE 4. *Frequency by decade of Aschoff bodies (AB) in necropsy and surgical patients with pure mitral regurgitation with or without dysfunction of other cardiac valves.*

meaningful (figs. 2 and 3). Thus, among our 206 necropsy patients with mitral stenosis, with or without other valve lesions, nine (4%) had Aschoff bodies, whereas among 390 surgical patients with mitral stenosis in whom left atrial appendage or papillary muscle or both were examined, 44 (11%) had Aschoff bodies ($P < 0.01$) (fig. 2). Because Aschoff bodies are observed infrequently in papillary muscle, the most meaningful comparison between the necropsy and surgical groups is made by comparing only the patients in whom left atrium was examined histologically. Thus, of the 206 necropsy patients with mitral stenosis, 9 (4%) had Aschoff bodies in the wall of left atrium, whereas of the 192 surgical patients with mitral stenosis, 40 (21%) had Aschoff bodies in the left atrium ($P < 0.01$) (fig. 2). The explanation for the difference in frequency (4% versus 21%) of Aschoff bodies in the necropsy and surgical group is uncertain. The average age of the necropsy and surgical patients, however, is different. The 206 necropsy patients with mitral stenosis, with or without other valve lesions, averaged 47 years of age (range 21–85), and the 192 surgical patients who underwent mitral commissurotomy for mitral stenosis aged 38 years of age (range 7–67) ($P < 0.01$) (fig. 3).

Aschoff bodies are significantly more frequent in patients with mitral stenosis than in patients with pure mitral regurgitation. Thus, of 95 necropsy patients examined who had pure mitral regurgitation, with or without dysfunction of one or more other cardiac valves, only one (1%) had Aschoff bodies (figs. 2 and 4), whereas of 206 necropsy patients with mitral stenosis, with or without dysfunction of one or more other cardiac valves, 9 (4%) had Aschoff bodies (fig. 2).

Among our 11 patients with Aschoff bodies at necropsy, nine had good historical evidence in the past of acute rheumatic fever. Although we are aware that historical evidence always represents "soft" data, the frequency of a positive history of acute rheumatic fever is strikingly different between patients with mitral valve disease compared to those with aortic valve disease. Among our 192 patients with clinically isolated aortic stenosis (table 2), only 12% had a history compatible with acute rheumatic fever. In contrast, of our 206 patients with mitral stenosis, with or without dysfunction of one or more other cardiac valves, 72% had a positive history of acute rheumatic fever. Thus, in general, *among patients with chronic valvular heart disease,* a positive history of acute rheumatic fever indicates a diffuse anatomic lesion of the mitral valve. The anatomic lesion, however, may or may not be of functional significance.

References

1. Aschoff L: Zur Myocarditisfrage, Verhandl. deutsch path Gesellsch **8**: 46, 1904
2. Rothschild MA, Kugel MA, Gross L: Incidence and significance of active infection in cases of rheumatic cardiovalvular disease during the various age periods. Am Heart J **9**: 586, 1934
3. McKeown F: The pathology of rheumatic fever. Ulester Med J **14**: 97, 1945
4. Pinniger JL: The left auricular appendage in mitral stenosis. St Thomas Hospital Reports **7**: 54, 1951
5. Waaler E: Study of auricular appendage in mitral stenosis. Acta Pathol Micro Scand Suppl **93**: 211, 1952
6. McKeown F: Left auricular appendage in mitral stenosis. Br Heart J **15**: 433, 1953
7. Decker JP, Hawn CVZ, Robbins SL: Rheumatic "activity" as judged by the presence of Aschoff bodies in auricular appendages of patients with mitral stenosis. I. Anatomic aspects. Circulation **8**: 161, 1953
8. Thomas WA, Averill JH, Castleman B, Bland EF: The significance of Aschoff bodies in the left atrial appendage. A comparison of 40 biopsies removed during mitral commissurotomy with autopsy material from 40 patients dying with fulminating rheumatic fever. N Engl J Med **249**: 761, 1953
9. Luse S, Rusted IE, Edwards JE: Aschoff bodies in surgically resected left auricular appendages and elsewhere in heart in mitral stenosis. Lab Invest **3**: 483, 1954
10. Tedeschi CG, Wagner BM, Pani KC: Studies in rheumatic fever. I. The clinical significance of the Aschoff body based on morphologic observations. AMA Arch Pathol **60**: 408, 1955
11. Lannigan R: The rheumatic process in the left auricular appendage. J Pathol Bacteriol **77**: 49, 1959
12. Ruebner BH, Boitnott JK: The frequency of Aschoff bodies in atrial appendages of patients with mitral stenosis. Relationship to age, atrial thrombosis, and season. Circulation **23**: 550, 1961
13. Virmani R, Roberts WC: Aschoff bodies in operatively excised atrial appendages and in papillary muscles. Frequency and clinical significance. Circulation **55**: 559, 1977
14. Saphir O: The Aschoff nodule. Am J Clin Pathol **31**: 534, 1959
15. Mortimer EA Jr: Control of rheumatic fever: How are we doing? JAMA **237**: 1720, 1977

Calcific Deposits in Stenotic Mitral Valves

Extent and Relation to Age, Sex, Degree of Stenosis, Cardiac Rhythm, Previous Commissurotomy and Left Atrial Body Thrombus from Study of 164 Operatively-Excised Valves

ANTHONY S. LACHMAN, M.B., AND WILLIAM C. ROBERTS, M.D.

SUMMARY The presence or absence and the extent of calcific deposits in excised stenotic mitral valves was determined by radiographs of the excised valve in 164 patients aged 26 to 72 years. The extent of the mitral calcific deposits was determined by the percent of the valvular circumference containing the deposits = grade 0 (14 patients); grade I = < 25% (43 patients); grade II = 25–50% (34 patients); grade III = 51–75% (39 patients); and grade IV = > 75% (34 patients). The amount of calcific deposits in the stenotic mitral valves correlated with sex and with the mean diastolic pressure gradient across the mitral valve ($P < 0.05$), but it did not correlate with the patient's age, cardiac rhythm, pulmonary arterial or pulmonary arterial wedge pressure, previous mitral commissurotomy, presence of thrombus in the body of left atrium or the presence of disease of one or more other cardiac valves.

AMONG PATIENTS WITH MITRAL STENOSIS, we know that calcific deposits in the mitral leaflets are common, a higher percentage of men have the deposits in their stenotic valves than do women, the results of commissurotomy are less satisfactory in those with noncalcified compared to those with calcified mitral valves, and the presence of calcific deposits usually necessitates the performance of valve replacement. We do not know whether calcific deposits in stenotic mitral valves and age are correlated. Furthermore, the relationship between the presence of, or the degree of mitral calcific deposits and the degree of mitral stenosis or other clinical parameters has not been investigated. The present report, therefore, attempts to fill in these voids by summarizing observations in 164 patients in whom mitral valve replacement was performed because of mitral stenosis. Calcium in the excised valve was determined qualitatively and quantitatively by radiography of the excised valve itself. Previous studies have relied on the judgment of the surgeon at operation, or preoperative routine roentgenography, fluoroscopy, or tomography for identification and quantification of calcific deposits in stenotic mitral valves.

Materials and Methods

The patients included in this study were derived from review of photographs of mitral valves excised at the National Heart, Lung, and Blood Institute from 1963 through 1976. Photographs were taken routinely of all excised valves during this period. A total of 293 patients underwent mitral valve replacement for mitral stenosis during this period. Of this number, unsectioned stenotic mitral valves were available for re-examination in 164 patients and these 164 form the basis of this report. A radiograph was taken on each of these 164 operatively excised valves via a Field-Emission-Faxitron-X-ray unit at 35 KVP. The X-ray beam was directed more or less perpendicular to the valve orifice. The presence of and the amount of calcium was determined by examination of the single radiograph of each excised

mitral valve. The amount of calcium in each valve was graded by the percent of circumference of the valve orifice occupied by calcium as follows: grade 0, no calcium; grade I, <25% of the circumference; grade II, 25–50%; grade III, 51–75%; and grade IV, >75%.

The degree of mitral stenosis and other clinical data were obtained from review of medical records. Mitral stenosis was confirmed by cardiac catheterization in all 164 patients. χ^2 tests were used on most of the two-way comparisons, and a distribution-free test for altered alternatives was used to compare the left atrial–left ventricular gradient to the degree of mitral valve calcium.

Results

The results are summarized in tables 1–5 and photographs of excised valves and radiographs of them are shown in figures 1–14. The 164 patients ranged in age from 26 to 72 years (median 51). The mean age of the 101 women was 52 years and for the 63 men, 48 years ($P < 0.05$). The amount of calcific deposits in the stenotic mitral valves did not correlate with age (table 1). Of the 91 patients with absent or light (grades 0, I, or II) calcific deposits, 41 (45%) were less than age 51 and 50 (55%) were greater than age 50; of the 73 patients with heavy (grades III or IV) calcific deposits, 37 (51%) were less than age 51 and 36 (49%) were greater than age 50. Of the total 164 patients, 78 (48%) were less than age 51 and 86 (52%) were greater than age 50.

The amount of calcific deposits in the stenotic mitral valves did correlate with sex (table 1). Of the 73 patients with heavy calcific deposits, 34 (47%) were men and 39 (53%) were women; of the 91 patients with absent or light calcific deposits, 29 (32%) were men, and 62 (68%) were women ($P < 0.05$). Of the 78 patients less than 51 years of age, 23 (61%) of the 38 men and 14 (35%) of the women had heavy calcific deposits ($P < 0.05$). Of the 15 patients less than age 41 with heavy calcific deposits, only 3 (20%) were women and 12 (80%) were men ($P < 0.05$). Of the 63 men, 20 (32%) had grade IV calcific deposits, and of the 101 women only 14 (14%) had similar sized deposits ($P < 0.05$). Furthermore, only 4 (6%) of the 63 men had no calcific deposits, whereas 10 (10%) of the 101 women had absent calcific deposits ($P < 0.05$).

From the Pathology Branch, National Heart, Lung, and Blood Institute, National Institutes of Health, Bethesda, Maryland.

Address for reprints: Dr. William C. Roberts, Building 10A, Room 3E-30, National Institutes of Health, Bethesda, Maryland 20014.

Received August 31, 1977; revision accepted October 31, 1977.

Table 1. *Calcific Deposits in Stenotic Mitral Valves: Amount of Calcium Related to Age and Sex*

Amount of Calcium	Ages (years)										Totals
	25-40		41-50		51-60		61-75		Subtotals		
	M	F	M	F	M	F	M	F	M	F	M + F
0	0	2	1	3	3	5	0	0	4	10	14 (8%)
I	3	7	4	6	5	11	1	6	13	30	43 (26%)
II	3	1	4	7	4	7	1	7	12	22	34 (21%)
III	3	3	5	8	4	9	2	5	14	25	39 (24%)
IV	9	0	6	3	4	7	1	4	20	14	34 (21%)
Totals	18	13	20	27	20	39	5	22	63	101	164 (100%)

Table 2. *Calcific Deposits in Stenotic Mitral Valves: Relation Between Valve Gradient and Sex*

Sex	Left atrial–Left ventricular mean diastolic gradient (mm Hg)			
	< 7.5	7.5 - 15	> 15	Totals
Males	4 (7%)	38 (60%)	21 (33%)	63 (100%)
Females	19 (19%)	46 (45%)	36 (36%)	101 (100%)
Totals	23 (14%)	84 (51%)	57 (35%)	164 (100%)

Table 4. *Calcific Deposits in Stenotic Mitral Valves: Amount of Calcium Related to Cardiac Rhythm*

Amount of Calcium	Sinus Rhythm	Atrial Fibrillation	Total
0	4 (29%)	10 (71%)	14
I	11 (26%)	32 (74%)	43
II	5 (15%)	29 (85%)	34
III	6 (15%)	33 (85%)	39
IV	12 (35%)	22 (65%)	34
Totals	38 (23%)	126 (77%)	164

Table 3. *Calcific Deposits in Stenotic Mitral Valves: Amount of Calcium Related to Mitral Valve Gradient*

Amount of Calcium	Mean Diastolic Pressure Gradient (in mm Hg) Between Left Atrium and Left Ventricle			
	< 7.5	7.5 - 15	> 15	Total
0	6	6	2	14
I	11	24	8	43
II	4	19	11	34
III	2	15	22	39
IV	0	20	14	34
Totals	23	84	57	164

Table 5. *Calcific Deposits in Stenotic Mitral Valves: Amount of Calcium Related Both to Left Atrial Body Thrombus and to Cardiac Rhythm*

Amount of Calcium	Left Atrial Thrombus	Sinus Rhythm	Atrial Fibrillation
0	1	0	1
I	4	1	3
II	7	1	6
III	7	0	7
IV	8	4	4
Totals	27	6	21

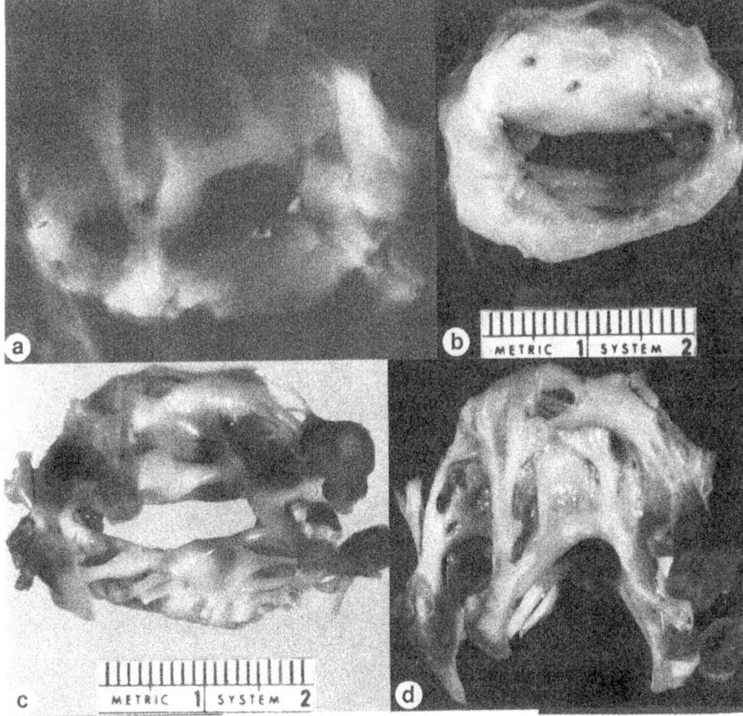

Figure 1. *Clinical data on each of the patients whose mitral valves are illustrated in this and the following figures are summarized in table 7. a) Radiograph. b) View from left atrium. c and d) View from left ventricle showing orifice in c and anterior leaflet and attached chordae tendineae in d.*

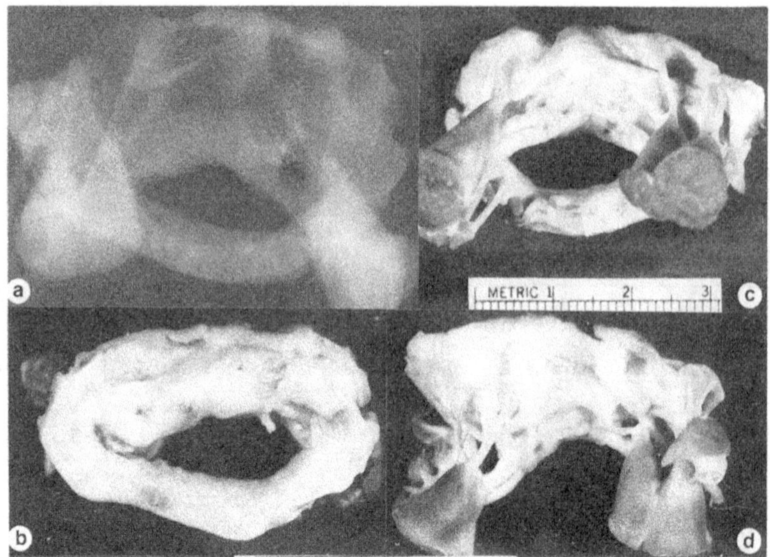

FIGURE 2. a) *Radiograph.* b) *View from left atrium.* c *and* d) *Views from left ventricle showing mitral orifice in* c *and anterior mitral leaflet in* d.

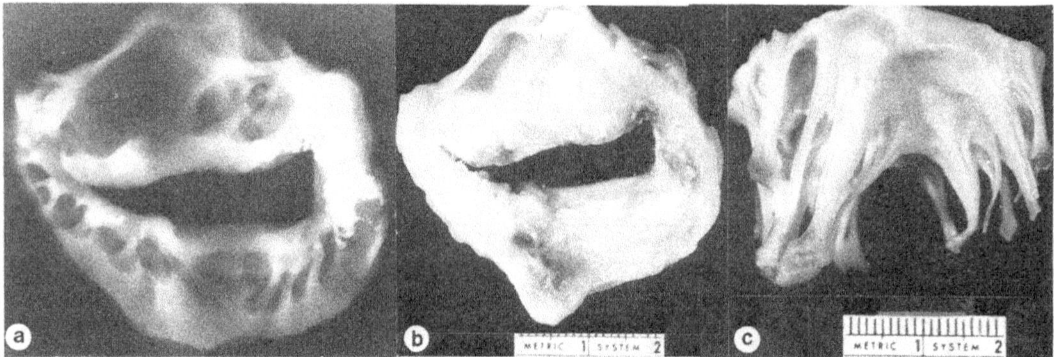

FIGURE 3. a) *Radiograph.* b) *View from left atrium.* c) *View of anterior leaflet from left ventricular aspect.*

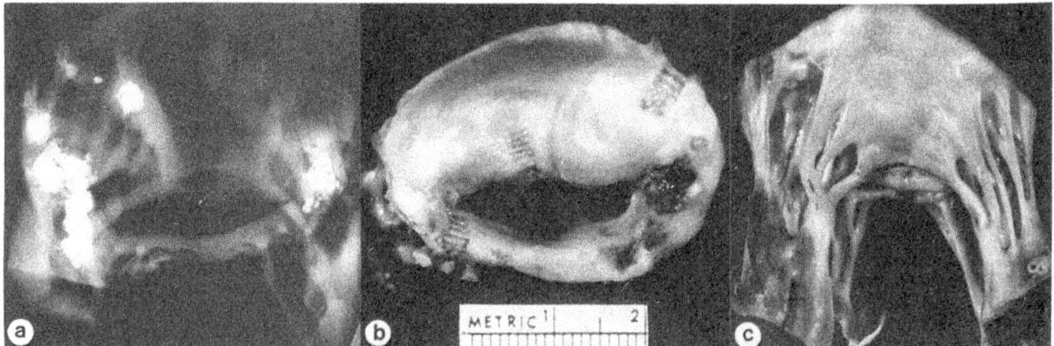

FIGURE 4. a) *Radiograph.* b) *View from left atrium.* c) *View of anterior leaflet from left ventricular aspect.*

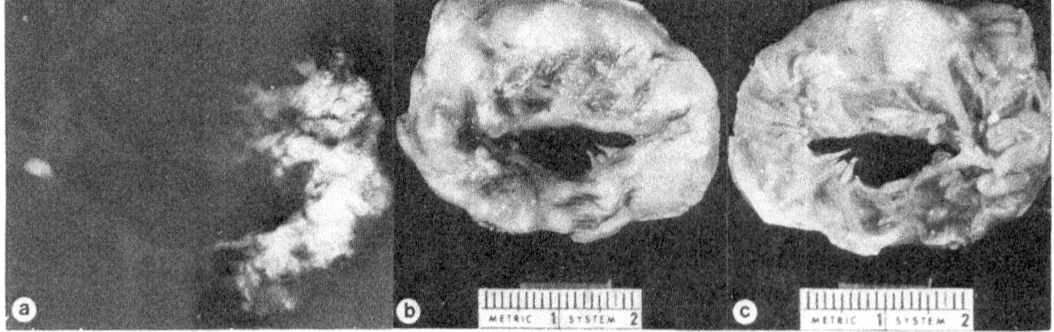

FIGURE 5. a) *Radiograph.* b) *View from left atrium.* c) *View from left ventricle after chordae tendineae were excised.*

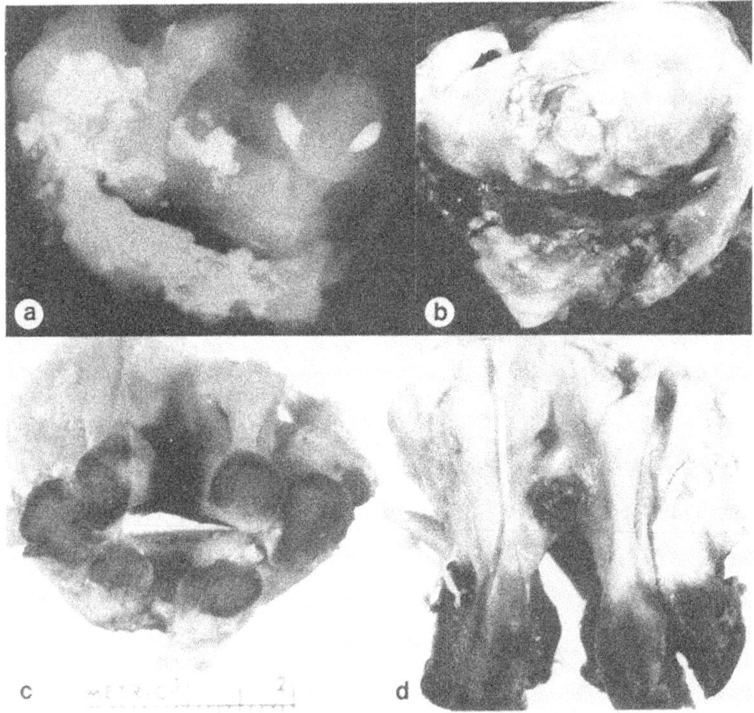

FIGURE 6. a) *Radiograph.* b) *View from left atrium.* c *and* d) *View of orifice* (c) *and anterior mitral leaflet* (d) *from left ventricular aspect.*

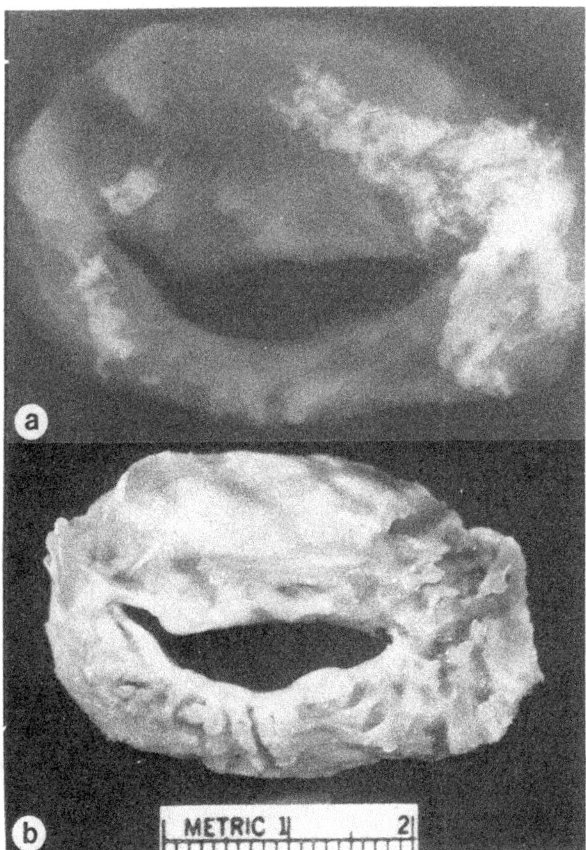

FIGURE 7. a) *Radiograph.* b) *View from left ventricular aspect after excision of the chordae tendineae.*

The *severity of the mitral stenosis* is summarized in tables 2 and 3 and in figure 15. The left atrial (or pulmonary arterial wedge) to left ventricular mean diastolic gradient in the 164 patients ranged from 4–30 mm Hg (avg 13.8 mm Hg). This gradient was identical in both men and women (13.8 mm Hg). Of the 164 patients, the gradients were greater than 15 in 57 (35%), between 7.5–15 in 84 (51%) and less than 7.5 in 23 (14%). The percent of men and women with gradients greater than 15 mm Hg was similar (33 and 36% respectively). Only four (6%) of the 63 men and 19 (19%) of the 101 women, however, had gradients less than 7.5 mm Hg ($P < 0.05$).

The degree of mitral stenosis did correlate with the amount of calcium present in the mitral leaflets (fig. 15). The left atrial to left ventricular mean diastolic gradient in the 57 patients with absent or grade I mitral calcific deposits averaged 10.7 mm Hg, whereas this gradient in the 73 patients with grade III or IV calcium averaged 16.4 mm Hg ($P < 0.01$) (fig. 15). This gradient in the 34 patients with grade II mitral calcium was midway between (13.5 mm Hg). Among the 57 patients with left atrial to left ventricular mean diastolic pressure gradients greater than 15 mm Hg, 36 (63%) had grade III or IV calcific deposits whereas only two (3%) had no calcific deposits ($P < 0.01$). Of the 23 patients with pressure gradients less than 7.5 mm Hg, only two (9%) had heavy (grade III or IV) calcific deposits, whereas 21 (91%) had absent or light (grades 0, I or II) calcific deposits ($P < 0.01$). Among the 84 patients with gradients between 7.5 and 15 mm Hg, 49 (58%) had absent or light and 35 (42%) had heavy calcific deposits.

Neither the pulmonary arterial systolic nor the pulmonary wedge mean pressures (144 patients) (left atrial mean

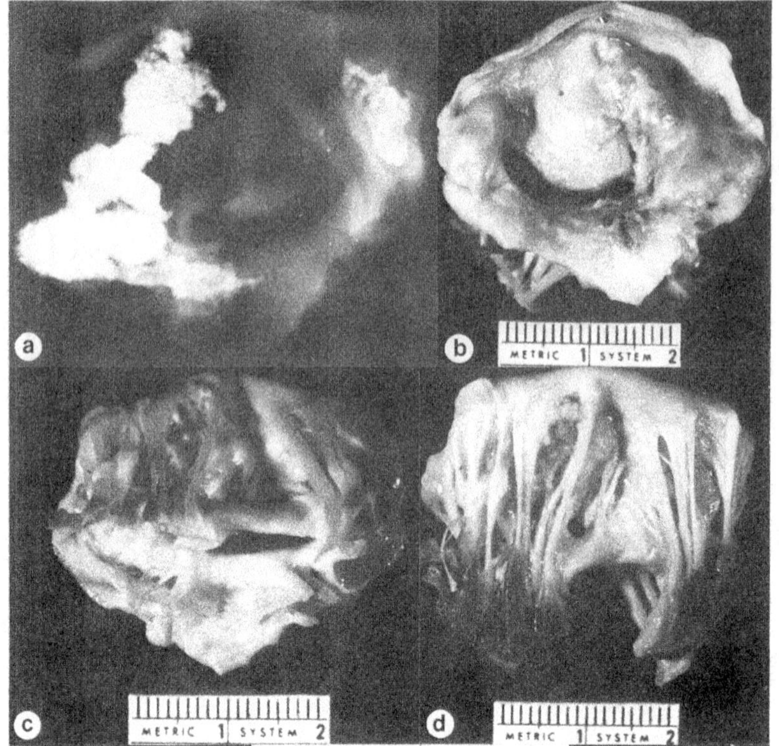

FIGURE 8. a) *Radiograph. Most of the calcific deposits are at and adjacent to the posteromedial commissure.* b) *View from left atrium.* c and d) *Views from left ventrical aspect showing the orifice* (c) *and anterior mitral leaflet* (d).

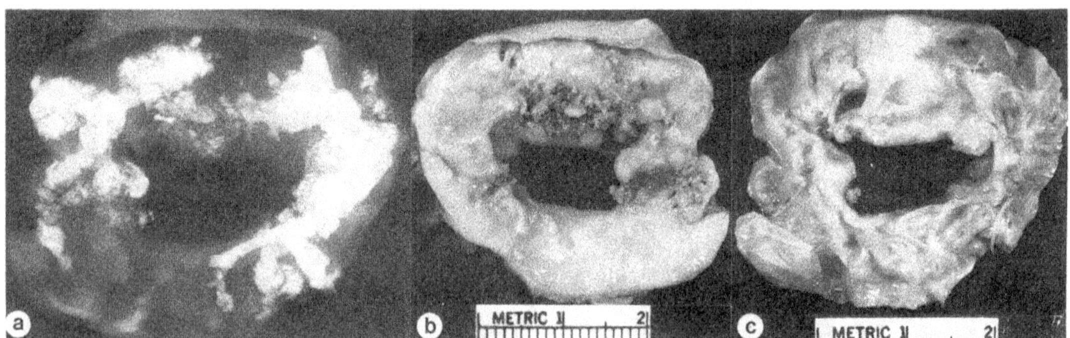

FIGURE 9. a) *Radiograph.* b) *View from left atrium.* c) *View from left ventricle.*

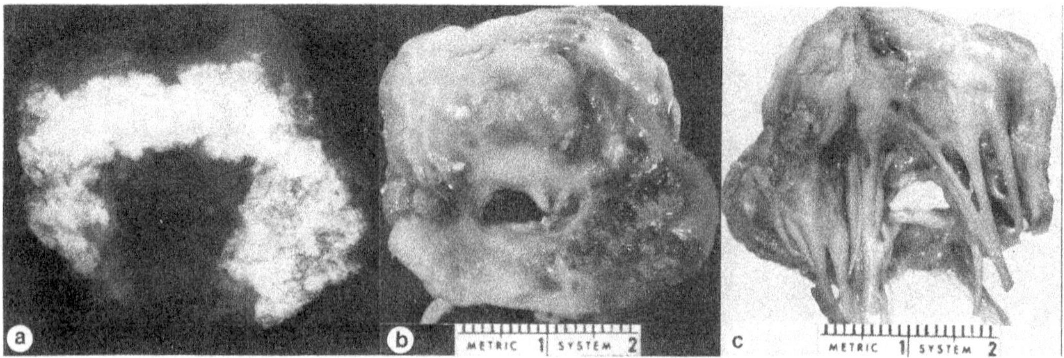

FIGURE 10. a) *Radiograph.* b) *View from left atrium.* c) *View from left ventricle.*

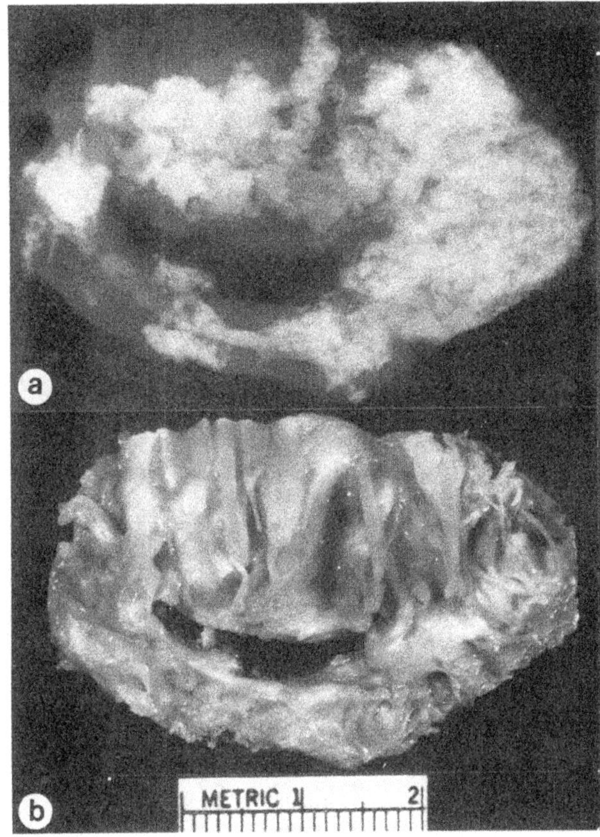

FIGURE 11. a) *Radiograph.* b) *View from left ventricle after excision of most chordae tendineae.*

pressure in 20 patients) correlated with the amount of mitral calcific deposits. Of the 162 patients with recorded pulmonary arterial systolic pressures, 50 (31%) were greater than 60 mm Hg, 54 (33%) were 45 to 60, 51 (32%) were 30 to 44, and only seven (4%) were normal (< 30 mm Hg). The pulmonary arterial wedge or left atrial mean pressures were greater than 25 mm Hg in 87 (53%) patients, between 12.5 and 25 mm Hg in 74 (45%) and less than 12.5 in four (3%) patients. The mitral valve area index decreased as the amount of the mitral calcific deposits increased.

Of the 164 patients before valve replacement, 38 (30%)

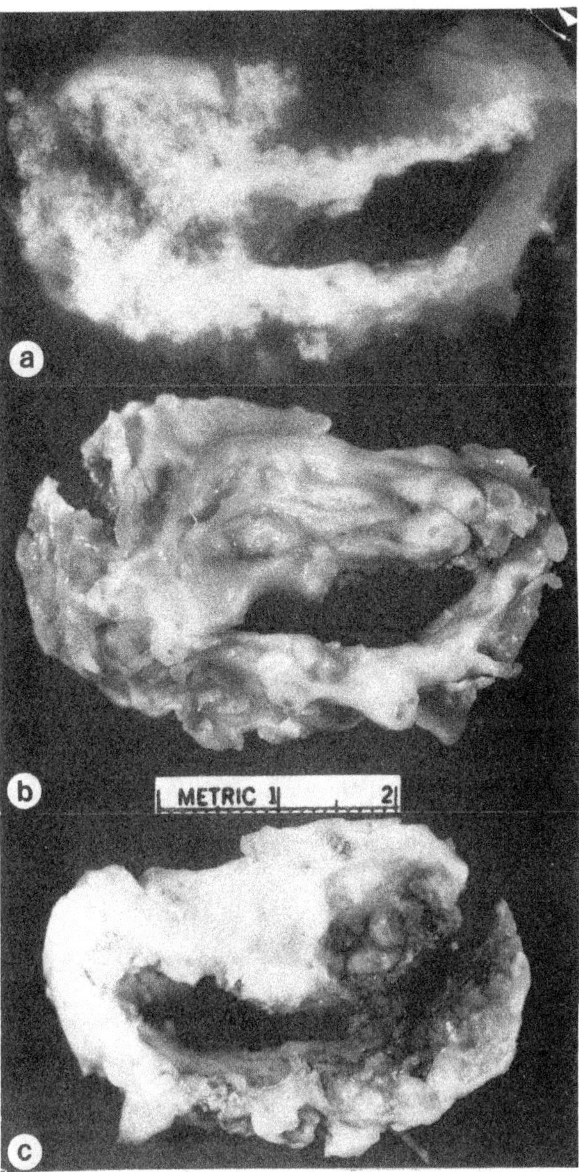

FIGURE 13. a) *Radiograph.* b) *View from left ventricle. The greatest amount of calcium is in the area of the posteromedial commissure.* c) *View from left atrial aspect.*

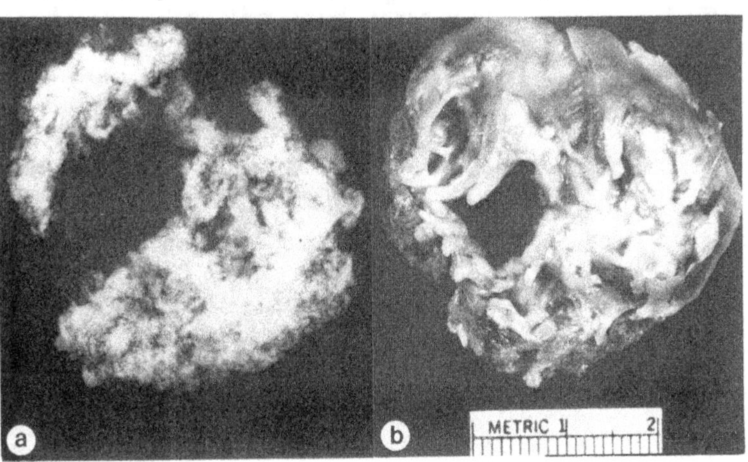

FIGURE 12. a) *Radiograph.* b) *View from left ventricular aspect after excision of most chordae tendineae.*

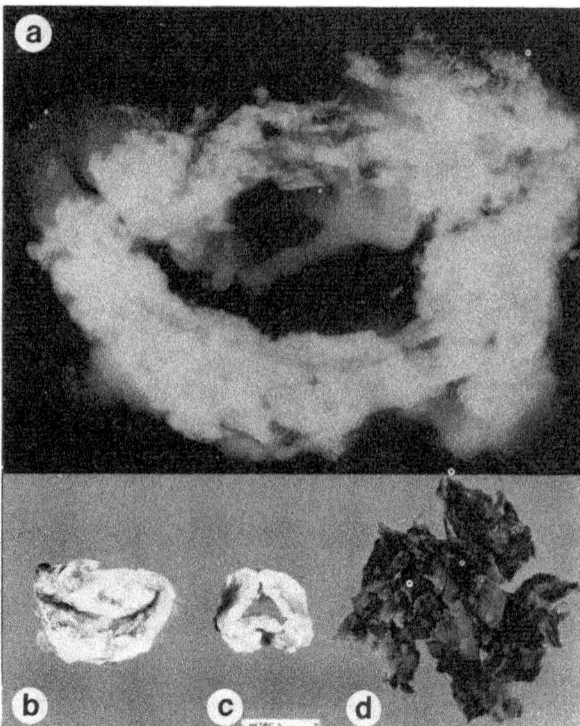

FIGURE 14. a) *Radiograph. Calcium extends around the entire 360° of the orifice.* b) *Mitral valve from left atrium.* c) *Excised, three-cuspid aortic valve with fusion of each of the 3 commissures.* d) *Thrombus excised from the body of left atrium.*

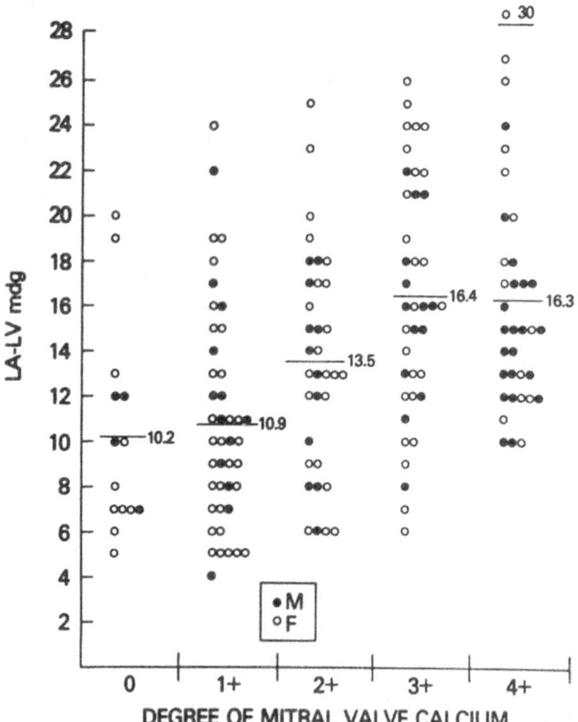

FIGURE 15. *Relation between left atrial (LA)-left ventricular (LV) mean diastolic gradient (mdg) and degree of mitral valve calcium.*

TABLE 6. *Calcific Deposits in Stenotic Mitral Valves: Amount of Calcium Related to Previous Mitral Commissurotomy (MC)*

Amount of Calcium	+ MC	O MC	Totals
0	6 (46%)	9 (64%)	14
I	18 (42%)	25 (58%)	43
II	11 (32%)	23 (68%)	34
III	14 (36%)	25 (64%)	39
IV	12 (35%)	22 (65%)	34
Totals	61 (37%)	103 (63%)	164

were in sinus rhythm and 126 (70%) were in chronic atrial fibrillation (table 4). The ages of the patients in sinus rhythm ranged from 33–68 years (avg. 47) and that of the 126 patients in atrial fibrillation, from 26–72 years (avg. 54) ($P < 0.05$). The rhythm, however, did not correlate with the amount of calcium in the stenotic mitral valves. Of the 126 patients in atrial fibrillation, 55 (44%) had heavy calcific deposits and of the 38 patients in sinus rhythm 18 (47%) had heavy calcific deposits.

The presence of *thrombus in the body of the left atrium* did not correlate with the amount of calcium in the stenotic mitral valves (table 5).

No relationship was found between the amount of mitral valve calcium and *previous mitral commissurotomy* (table 6). Of the 164 patients, 61 (37%) had mitral commissurotomy from 6 months to 19 years before mitral valve replacement.

No correlation was found between the amount of mitral calcium and the *presence of other cardiac valve lesions.* Of the 164 patients, 79 (48%) had isolated mitral stenosis with or without mitral regurgitation, and 85 (52%) patients had other valve lesions: aortic stenosis with or without aortic regurgitation in 47 patients (29%), pure aortic regurgitation in 30 (18%), and tricuspid stenosis with or without tricuspid regurgitation in 8 (5%). Pure tricuspid valve regurgitation was not included among the patients with associated valve lesions. In 59 (77%) of the 77 patients with associated aortic valve disease, aortic valve replacement also was carried out.

Comments

Clinical assessment of mitral calcific deposits has been made previously utilizing fluoroscopy, tomography, and angiocardiography.[1-3] While each could indicate the presence or absence of such deposits, these methods failed to quantify them. Radiography of the excised mitral valve allows accurate assessment of the amount of mitral calcific deposits. Wooley and associates[4] described the location and extent of such deposits in 23 patients with mitral stenosis, but they did not relate the morphologic changes to clinical or hemodynamic factors. Our method of expressing the degree of calcific deposits in this valve as a percentage of the valve orifice circumference provides a means of relating the morphological changes to the hemodynamic data.

The present study of 164 patients aged 26 to 72 years shows that the amount of calcific deposits in stenotic mitral valves correlated with *sex* and with the *mean diastolic pressure gradient* across the mitral valve, but not with the patient's age, cardiac rhythm, main pulmonary arterial or pulmonary arterial wedge pressure, previous mitral com-

TABLE 7. *Clinical Data in the 14 Patients Whose Mitral Valves Are Illustrated in Figures 1-14*

Fig. no.	Surgical number	MV Ca++ 1+-4+	Age (yrs.)	Sex	MVC in past	PAW-LV mdg (mm Hg)	PA Pressure (mm Hg) s/d	Rhythm SR	AF	LV-SA psg (mm Hg)	LA Body Thr	MR (0-4+) by LV cine
1	S73-5005	1+	40	F	0	11	70/40	0	+	0	0	2+
2	S67-686	1+	40	F	+	13	50/18	0	+	0	0	3+
3	S75-5138	2+	41	F	0	7	32/14	0	+	0	0	3+
4	S70-3120	2+	55	F	0	9	28/12	0	+	0	0	2+
5	S76-28	2+	58	M	+	12	40/20	0	+	0	0	1+
6	S71-3012	3+	50	F	0	22	75/22	0	+	0	+	—
7	S67-4943	3+	50	M	0	16	55/30	0	+	20	0	1+
8	S76-52	3+	50	F	0	16	60/30	0	+	0	+	1+
9	S67-3587	4+	45	F	0	24	110/52	+	0	0	0	1+
10	S75-5128	4+	33	M	0	15	120/60	+	0	0	0	3+
11	S67-867	4+	53	F	0	26	88/45	+	0	0	+	1+
12	S70-3021	4+	26	M	0	15	55/27	0	+	0	0	1+
13	S66-4095	4+	43	M	0	23	61/37	+	0	7	0	2+
14	S70-3005	4+	37	M	+	9	95/45	+	0	34	+	—

Abbreviations: AF = atrial fibrillation; Ca++ = calcium; F = female; Hg = mercury; M = male; mdg = mean diastolic gradient; mm = millimeters; MR = mitral regurgitation; MV = mitral valve; MVC = mitral valve commissurotomy; LA = left atrium; LV = left ventricle; PA = pulmonary artery; PAW = pulmonary artery wedge; psg = peak systolic gradient; SA = systemic artery; s/d = systolic/diastolic; SR = sinus rhythm; and Thr = thrombus.

missurotomy, presence of thrombus in the body of left atrium or the presence of disease in one or more other cardiac valves.

Men tend to have heavier calcific deposits in stenotic mitral valves and at an earlier age than do women with the same hemodynamic lesion. Over twice as many men had extremely heavy (grade IV) mitral calcific deposits than women, whereas the opposite occurred in the patients with no mitral calcific deposits. Olesen and associates,[2] from study by tomography, also demonstrated a much higher frequency of calcific deposits in stenotic mitral valves of men compared to women (nearly 3 to 1), but quantitation of the amount of calcium was not determined. Kitchin and Turner[3] determined the presence or absence of mitral calcific deposits by palpation at commissurotomy or by preoperative radiography, and they too found a higher incidence of mitral calcific deposits in men, and they also found an increased incidence of calcific deposits in stenotic mitral valves in their older patients. Neither of the latter two studies, however, attempted to quantitate the amount of calcific deposits in these stenotic mitral valves. We did not find heavier mitral calcific deposits in our older patients compared to the younger patients.

The mean diastolic pressure gradient across the mitral valve in our patients increased as the amount of calcium in this valve increased. This correlation has not been provided previously. A similar correlation regarding calcific deposits in stenotic *aortic* valves has been noted previously.[5]

Surprisingly, 12 (35%) of the 34 patients with the heaviest (grade IV) mitral calcific deposits had sinus rhythm. Of the 91 patients with absent or light (grade I and II) calcific deposits, 71 (78%) had atrial fibrillation.

Previous commissurotomy did not correlate with the extent of calcific deposits observed in the excised stenotic mitral valves. Indeed, the percent of patients in each of the five grades of mitral calcific deposits was similar. Thus, mitral valve commissurotomy does not appear to increase mitral valve calcific deposits and furthermore, an earlier mitral commissurotomy does not indicate that commissurotomy cannot be performed a second time. In retrospect, possibly several of the 24 patients in this analysis who had absent (6 patients) or only grade 1 (18 patients) mitral calcific deposits could have had another mitral commissurotomy rather than valve replacement during the second cardiotomy. None of the 18 patients with only grade I calcific deposits by radiography of the excised valve had calcific deposits by radiography (any method) before valve replacement.

Acknowledgments

This study was made possible because the mitral valves had been excised intact and because hemodynamic studies had been performed on all patients preoperatively. Therefore, we are enormously indebted to Dr. Andrew G. Morrow who has virtually always excised cardiac valves at operation *intact* and has stressed the importance of doing so to his associates. To Dr. Stephen E. Epstein and earlier to Dr. Eugene Braunwald and their colleagues we are grateful for free access to the hemodynamic information in their patients. Ms. Barbara E. Winterrowd and Filippina Giacometti provided technical assistance. The gross anatomy photographs were taken by Mr. L. Kenzie Edwards and James R. Banks, Jr. Mr. H. Robert Baird, Laboratory of Statistical and Mathematical Methodolology, Division of Computer Research and Technology, NIH, provided the statistical analyses.

References

1. Wynn A: Gross calcification of the mitral valve. Br Heart J 15: 214, 1953
2. Olsen K, Dandoe E, Gudbjerg C: The higher incidence of valvular calcification in males than in females with mitral stenosis. Acta Medica Scand 177 (fasc. 1): 7, 1965
3. Kitchin A, Turner R: Calcification of the mitral valve. Results of valvotomy in 100 cases. Br Heart J 29: 137, 1967
4. Wooley CF, Baba N, Kilman J, Rayna J: Thrombotic calcific mitral stenosis: Morphology of the calcific mitral valve. Circulation 49: 1167, 1974
5. Glancy DL, Freed TA, O'Brien KP, Epstein SE: Calcium in the aortic valve. Roentgenologic and hemodynamic correlation in 148 patients. Ann Intern Med 71: 245, 1969

Mitral valve *commissurotomy* versus *replacement*

Considerations based on examination of operatively excised stenotic mitral valves

William C. Roberts, M.D.
Anthony S. Lachman, M.B., F.C.P. (S.A.)
Bethesda, Md.

Recently, we studied 164 operatively-excised stenotic mitral valves and by radiography of the excised valve quantitated the amount of calcific deposits in them.[1] Of the 164 stenotic valves, 14 had absent and 43 had minimal calcific deposits by x-ray of the excised valve. Of these 57 patients with absent or minimal calcific deposits, 37 had moderate to severe mitral regurgitation, and, therefore, clearly deserved mitral valve replacement. The remaining 20 had absent or minimal mitral regurgitation, absent or minimal calcific deposits, and mitral valve replacement, nevertheless, was carried out. This report focuses on these latter 20 patients to ask if mitral valve replacement was preferable to mitral valve commissurotomy.

Patients studied

Of the 20 patients, 19 underwent mitral valve replacement from 1970 to 1976 and one in 1967. The mitral valve operations on these 20 patients during the 8 years were done by five different surgeons (see Acknowledgment). Certain clinical and morphologic features in the 20 patients are summarized in Table I and morphologic and radiographic features of the excised mitral valves are illustrated in Figs. 1 to 5. A radiograph was taken of each of the excised mitral valves via a Field-Emission-Faxitron x-ray unit at 35 KVP. No calcific deposits were present in the excised

From the Pathology Branch, National Heart, Lung, and Blood Institute, National Institutes of Health, Bethesda, Md.

Received for publication June 2, 1978.

Accepted for publication July 14, 1978.

Reprint requests to: Dr. William C. Roberts, Building 10A, Room 3E30, National Institutes of Health, Bethesda, Md. 20014.

valve in five patients and in the other 15, calcific deposits were trace, minimal, or mild and in no patient were they visible before operation by routine chest roentgenogram or by fluoroscopy.

The 20 patients ranged in age from 36 to 62 years (average, 52 years); 12 (60 per cent) were women and eight were men. Cardiac catheterization was carried out during the 2 months before mitral valve replacement in all 20 patients (Table I). The mean diastolic pressure gradients between pulmonary artery wedge and left ventricle ranged from 5 to 21 mm. Hg (average, 11.5 mm. Hg). The pulmonary arterial systolic pressures (19 patients) ranged from 32 to 75 mm. Hg (average, 50 mm. Hg). The mean pulmonary arterial wedge pressures ranged from 15 to 35 mm. Hg (average, 25 mm. Hg). In eight patients, a systolic pressure gradient was present between left ventricle and systemic artery and it ranged from 10 to 95 mm. Hg (average, 50 mm. Hg). The cardiac index ranged from 1.2 to 3.6 L./min./M.^{2} (average, 2.09 L./min./M.^{2}). Left ventricular angiography in 19 patients indicated minimal $(1+/4+)$ mitral regurgitation in 16 patients and no regurgitation in three patients. The one patient (No. 10, Table I) in whom left ventricular angiography was not performed had no precordial systolic murmur. Injection of contrast material into the aortic "root" in 18 patients indicated various degrees of aortic regurgitation in 14.

In addition to mitral valve replacement, the aortic valve was replaced in 12 (60 per cent) of the 20 patients and the tricuspid valve, in four (20 per cent), three of whom also had aortic valve replacement. The average mean diastolic pressure gradient between pulmonary arterial wedge posi-

Table I. Clinical and hemodynamic data in the 20 patients analyzed

Surgical Number	Age (yrs)	Sex	Interval MVC to MVR (yrs)	PAW-LV mdg* (mm. Hg)	PA* (s/d) (mm. Hg)	CI* (L./min. /M.²)	MR by LV cine* (0-4+)	MV Ca⁺⁺ by x-ray of excised valve (0+ 4+)	LV-SA PSG* (mm. Hg)	AR by AA cine* (0-4+)	AVR	TVR	Fig. No.
No previous mitral-valve commissurotomy													
1 67-3005	36	M	—	8	32/10	1.7	1+	1+	26	2+	+	0	—
2 70-3094	47	M	—	11	50/20	1.8	1+	1+	0	2+	+	0	—
3 70-3127	44	F	—	15	45/32	1.7	1+	1+	10	3+	+	+	—
4 72-4096	57	F	—	5	34/18	2.0	0	0	40	4+	+	0	—
5 73-5085	60	M	—	17	—	1.5	1+	1+	0	3+	+	0	—
6 74-5139	48	M	—	12	50/20	3.1	0	1+	50	3+	+	0	—
7 75-5067	52	F	—	21	60/30	2.3	1+	0	90	2+	+	+	—
8 75-5106	58	M	—	10	70/40	3.6	1+	0	0	0	0	0	1
9 76-28	58	M	—	12	40/20	2.3	1+	1+	0	0	0	0	—
Previous mitral-valve commissurotomy													
10 71-3125	59	F	17 & 14	11**	36/18	1.7	—***	1+	0	—	0	0	2
11 71-3136	62	F	15	11	48/23	2.6	1+	1+	0	1+	0	0	3
12 71-3144	61	F	19	10	70/35	3.4	1+	1+	0	1+	0	0	4
13 72-5003	64	F	10	15	75/35	1.2	0	1+	0	1+	0	0	—
14 73-5032	57	F	12	8	55/25	2.3	1+	1+	0	0	0	0	—
15 73-5071	49	M	18	10	50/20	2.2	1+	1+	95	2+	+	0	—
16 74-5047	47	M	2	14	45/24	2.5	1+	1+	0	2+	+	0	—
17 74-5156	36	F	8	7	40/20	1.0	1+	0	75	—	+	+	5
18 75-5162	43	F	15 & 8	10	55/25	1.7	1+	1+	0	0	0	+	
19 76-95	51	F	6	16	55/28	2.0	1+	1+	10	2+	+	0	—
20 76-99	42	F	4	7	32/15	1.2	1+	0	0	3+	+	0	—

*At cardiac catheterization performed during the 2 months before mitral valve replacement.

**Left atrial pressure.

***A precordial systolic murmur was absent.

Abbreviations: AA = ascending aorta; AR = aortic regurgitation; AVR = aortic valve replacement; CI = cardiac index; F = female; LA = left atrial; LV = left ventricular; M = male; mdg = mean diastolic gradient; MR = mitral regurgitation; MV = mitral valve; MVC = mitral valve commissurotomy; MVR = mitral valve replacement; PA = pulmonary arterial; PAW = pulmonary arterial wedge; PSG = peak systolic gradient; SA = systemic arterial; s/d = systolic/diastolic; TVR = tricuspid valve replacement.

tion and left ventricle in the patients who underwent aortic valve replacement was 11.9 mm. Hg, and in those in whom this valve was not replaced, it was 10.9 mm. Hg.

Of the 20 patients, 11 had had mitral commissurotomy from 2 to 19 years (average, 12 years) previously. Two patients (No. 10 and No. 18, Table I) had had two previous commissurotomies. The pulmonary arterial wedge to left ventricular mean diastolic pressure gradients in these 11 patients ranged from 7 to 16 mm. Hg (average, 10.8 mm. Hg), whereas this gradient in the nine patients without previous commissurotomy ranged from 5 to 21 mm. Hg (average, 12.3 mm. Hg).

Thrombus was found in the body of left atrium at the time of valve replacement in two patients (No. 10 and No. 18, Table I).

Comments

The absence of significant calcific deposits (as determined by radiography of the excised valve) and the absence of significant mitral regurgitation (as determined by left ventricular angiography) in the operatively-excised stenotic mitral valves described above raises the question as to whether mitral valve replacement in these 20 patients was preferable to commissurotomy. To answer this question the stenotic mitral valves in patients having only commissurotomy would have to be studied morphologically and radiographically in the same manner as the valves which were excised and replaced. Obviously, the non-excised valve cannot be examined in the same manner as the excised valve. Nevertheless, the ideal valve for mitral commissurotomy in the past has been considered to be the stenotic one

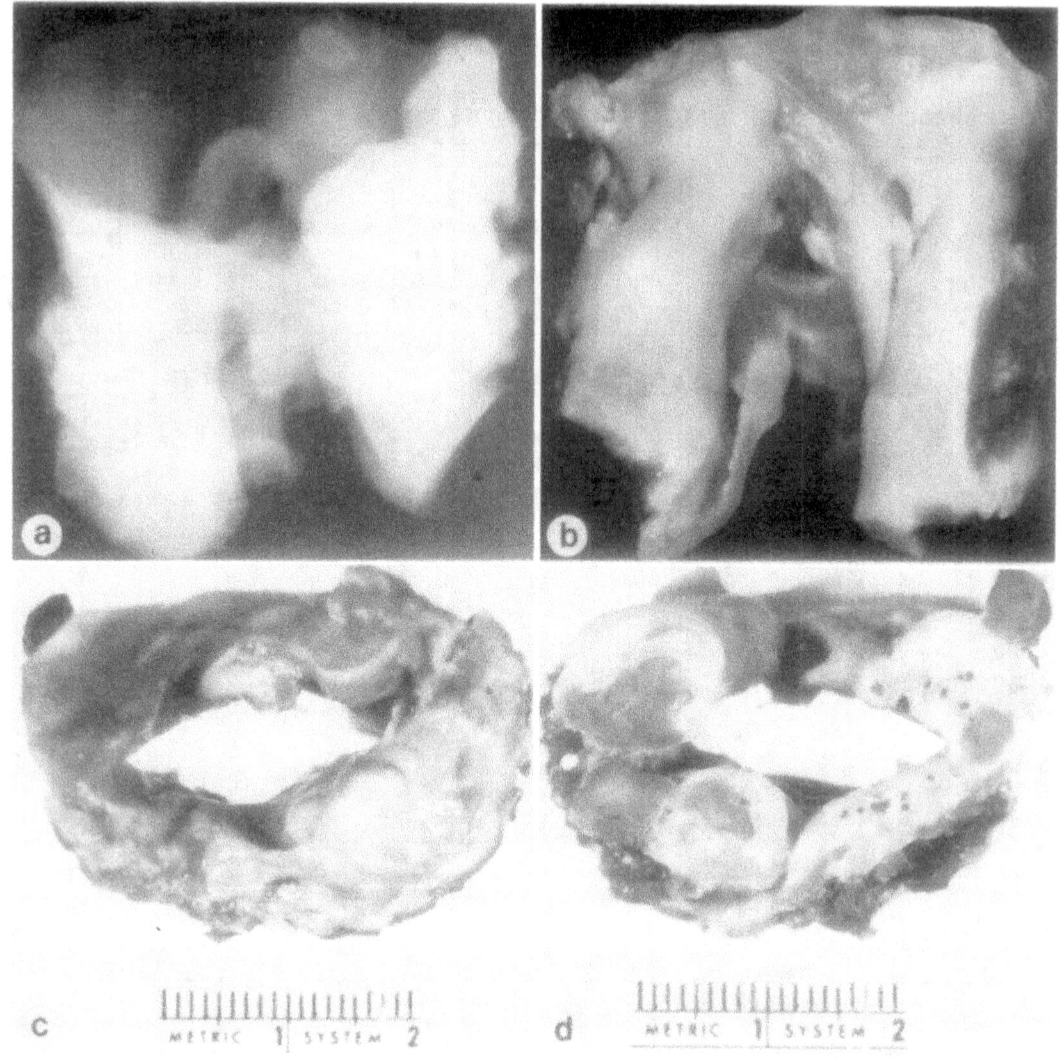

Fig. 1, a through d. Case No. 8 (Table 1). *a,* Radiograph showing no calcific deposits. *b,* View of anterior leaflet and papillary muscles from left ventricle. The papillary muscles are covered by thick fibrous tissue. *c,* View from left atrium. *d,* View of orifice from left ventricle again showing the thick fibrous tissue overlying the papillary muscles.

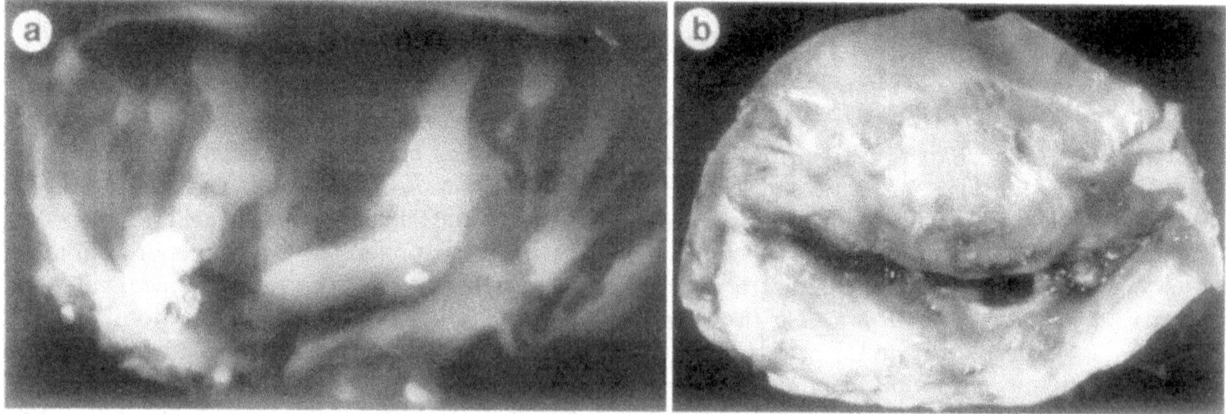

Fig. 2, a and b. Case No. 10 (Table I). *a,* Radiograph showing two calcific deposits. *b,* View from left atrium.

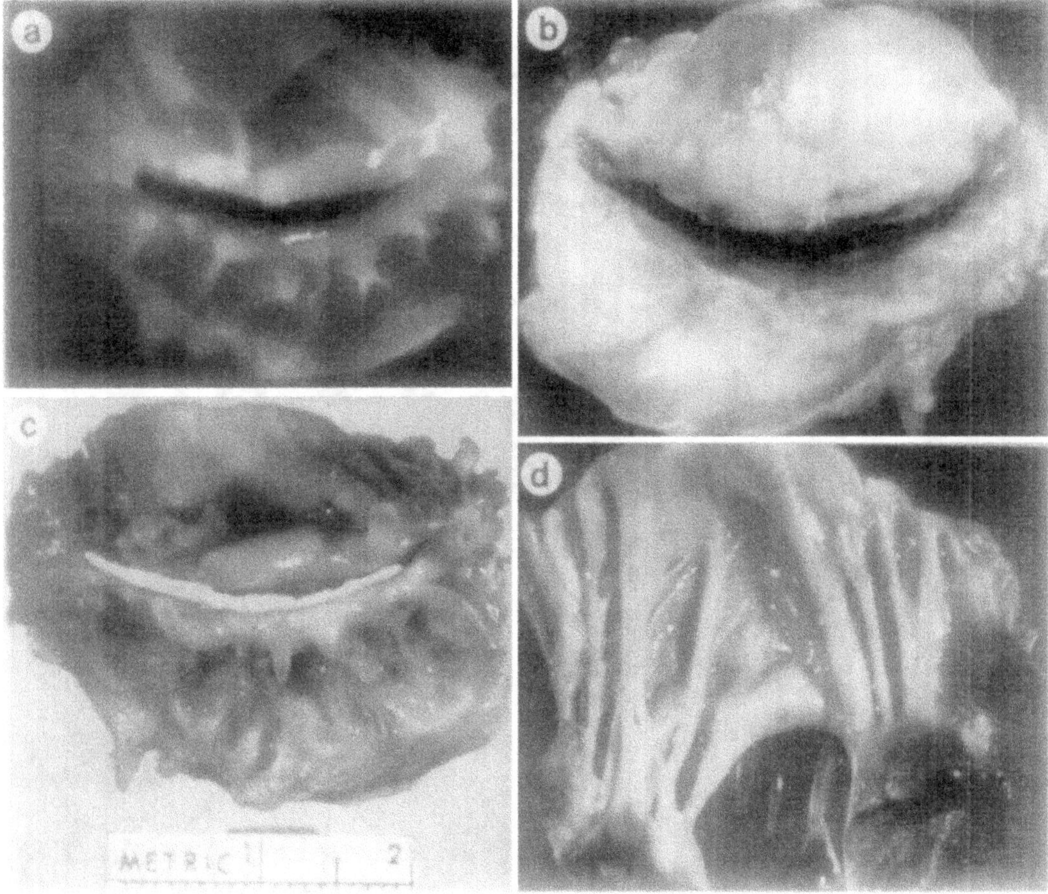

Fig. 3, a through **d**. Case No. 11 (Table I). *a*, Radiograph showing three minute calcific deposits. *b*, View from left atrium. *c*, View from left ventricle after excision of the chordae tendineae. *d*, View of anterior leaflet from left ventricle.

which is free of calcific deposits, free of significant mitral regurgitation, and mobile.[2-10] The excised mitral valves in the 20 patients analyzed here were free of calcific deposits by preoperative examination, and none had significant mitral regurgitation by preoperative evaluation. Mobility of the mitral valve at the time of valve replacement was described in the operative note in six of the 20 patients and in each mobility was limited, particularly so in four patients. Small calcific deposits in the mitral leaflets, however, were noted at operation in 10 patients; in three others, calcific deposits were noted to be absent, and in the remaining seven patients no mention was made in the operative note regarding their presence or absence. Radiography, however, of the excised valve disclosed no calcific deposits in five patients and minimal deposits in 15. In two of the patients stated to have calcific deposits in the mitral valve at operation, radiography of the

excised valve disclosed no calcific deposits, indicating that palpation and visual inspection is not always accurate with respect to calcific deposits.

It seems likely that all 20 patients analyzed here would have been acceptable candidates for mitral commissurotomy alone in the pre-valve replacement era. Why then was mitral valve replacement rather than commissurotomy carried out? One factor certainly was the fact *that one or more other valves were replaced.* Thirteen of the 20 patients also underwent replacement of the aortic or tricuspid valve or both. Under these circumstances, mitral replacement may be advisable rather than risk possible significant regurgitation or incomplete relief of the stenosis by mitral commissurotomy.

Another consideration was the fact that *cardiopulmonary bypass was utilized* in each patient. This procedure obviously allows visual

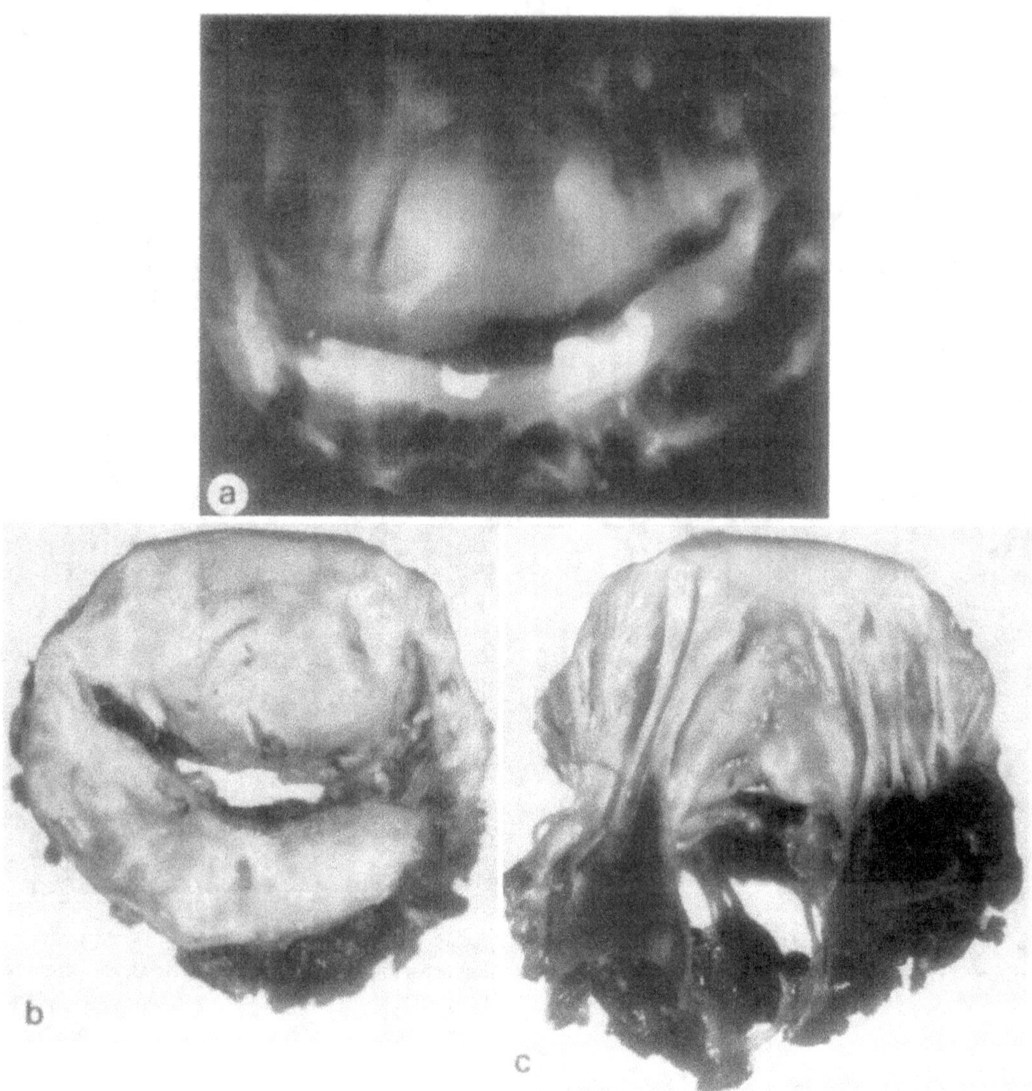

Fig. 4, a through c. Case No. 12 (Table I). *a*, Radiograph. *b*, View from left atrium. *c*, View of anterior leaflet and papillary muscles from left ventricle.

inspection of the valve, something not possible when commissurotomy was done as a "closed" procedure. We suspect that the visually inspected stenotic mitral valve is more frightening to the observer than is the stenotic valve which is only palpated. Thus, visual inspection alone, particularly when valve replacement is a reasonable and uncriticized option, may push the surgeon in some patients toward replacement rather than simple commissurotomy.

Another factor was *relatively little experience of some surgeons with mitral commissurotomy,* particularly as an open procedure, compared to valve replacement. Of the 20 study patients, 17 were operated upon by surgeons less than 40 years of age when the operation was done. The younger surgeons have had less experience with the commissurotomy procedure than with valve replacement, and consequently may feel more comfortable with the latter procedure.

Another factor was *displeasure with the attempted commissurotomy.* Three patients (No. 3, No. 4, and No. 6, Table I) had open mitral commissurotomy attempted but the surgeon was not satisfied with his results and valve replacement, therefore, was done.

And finally, *previous mitral valve commissurotomy* probably contributed to the decision. Eleven of the 20 patients had had at least one previous mitral commissurotomy. Examination of the

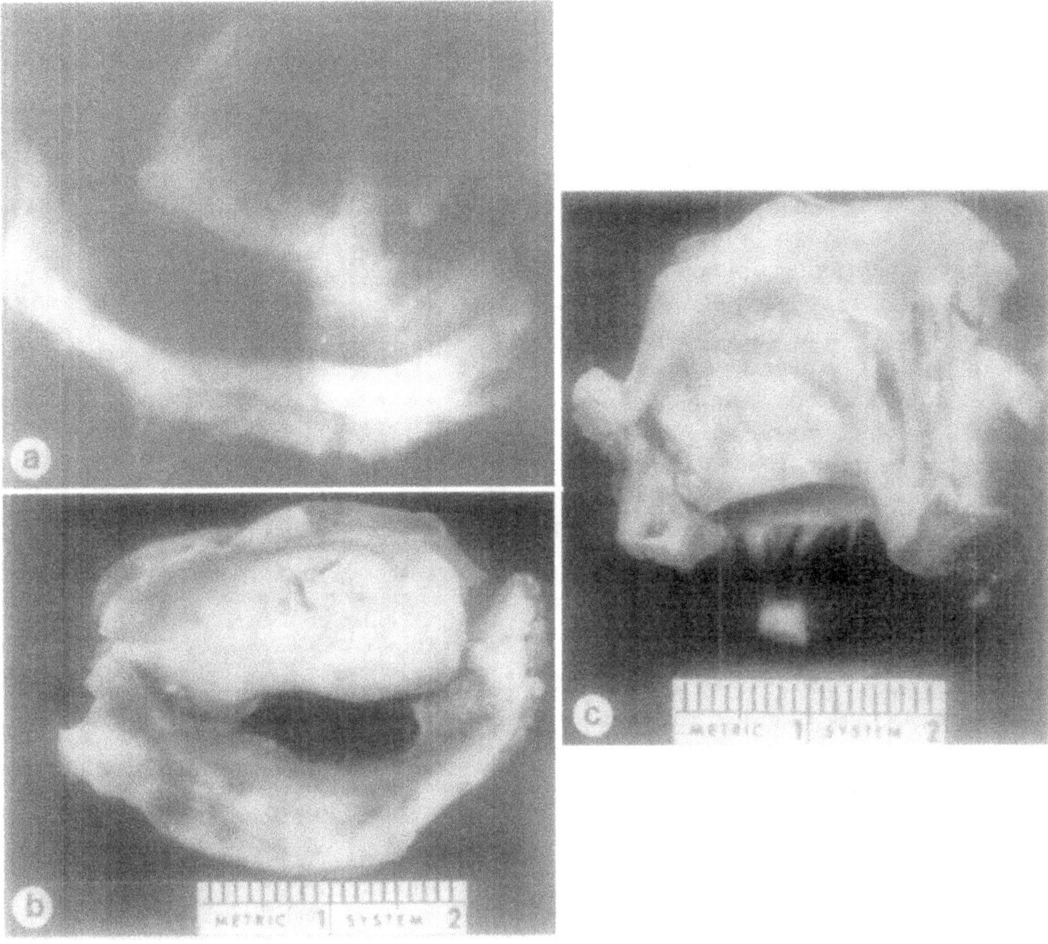

Fig. 5, a through **c.** Case No. 17 (Table I). *a,* Radiograph showing no calcific deposits. *b,* View from left atrium. *c,* View of anterior leaflet from left ventricle.

excised mitral valve in several of these 11 patients, however, showed no anatomic residua of the previous commissurotomy. Therefore, as is already recognized,[11] a mitral valve which has had one previous commissurotomy and later becomes severely stenotic again can, nevertheless, have another commissurotomy so long as calcific deposits are absent and mitral regurgitation is absent or is minimal.

Thus as emphasized recently by Spencer[12] "... the relative frequency of mitral valve reconstruction (i.e., commissurotomy) versus replacement will vary not only with the *experience* and *attitude* of the surgeon but with the *type of valve pathology seen*... a surgeon experienced and enthusiastic about reconstruction might perform commissurotomy in 95 per cent of cases if patients are referred for operation with relatively early disease, while a similar surgeon might find it necessary to perform replacement in over 30 per cent of cases if patients are referred only with far advanced disease and extensive calcification."[12] Nevertheless, the definition of "advanced disease" appears to be changing, but as yet there is insufficient information to know whether this apparent change will prove to be beneficial or detrimental to the patient.

Summary

Among 164 patients who underwent mitral valve replacement because of mitral stenosis (with or without mitral regurgitation) and had radiographs taken of their operatively excised mitral valves, 20 had absent or minimal calcific deposits in the excised valves and absent or minimal mitral regurgitation as determined, except for one patient, by left ventricular angiography preoperatively. This report focuses on these 20 patients to ask if mitral valve replacement was preferable to mitral valve commissurotomy. Although in the pre-valve replacement era, all 20 patients almost surely would have been considered good candidates for mitral commissurotomy, other factors, namely, the need to replace one or more other cardiac valves (13 patients), the utilization of cardiopulmonary bypass allowing visual inspection rather than simple palpation of the diseased mitral valve (all 20 patients), relatively little experience with mitral commissurotomy in four of the five surgeons (17 patients), displeasure with attempted commissurotomy (three patients), previous mitral commissurotomy (11 patients), and incorrect identification of mitral calcific deposits (two patients), each contributed in one or more patients to the final decision of replacement versus commissurotomy. Even though mitral commissurotomy has been in use for 30 years, the mere alternative of valve replacement may have altered somewhat the definition of the stenotic mitral valve previously considered ideal for mitral commissurotomy.

The authors are indebted to the five surgeons who operated on the 20 patients analyzed in this report. These surgeons and the number of patients operated on by them were the following: Charles L. McIntosh (7), Lawrence L. Michaelis (7), Andrew G. Morrow (3), Robert L. Reis (2), and Edward B. Stinson (1). We thank Dr. Andrew G. Morrow for reviewing the manuscript, and Dr. Stephen E. Epstein for free use of the hemodynamic data in the study patients.

REFERENCES

1. Lachman, A. S., and Roberts, W. C.: Calcific deposits in stenotic mitral valves. Extent and relationship to age, sex, degree of stenosis, cardiac rhythm, previous commissurotomy and left atrial body thrombus from study of 164 operatively-excised valves. Circulation 57:808, 1978.
2. Ellis, L. B., and Harken, D. E.: Closed valvuloplasty for mitral stenosis. A twelve-year follow-up study of 1571 patients, N. Engl. J. Med. 270:643, 1964.
3. Morrow, A. G., Harrison, D. C., Ross, J., Jr., Braunwald, N. S., Clark, W. D., and Ross, R. S.: The surgical management of mitral valve disease: A symposium on diagnostic methods, operative techniques and results. Combined Clinical Staff Conference at the National Institutes of Health, Ann. Intern. Med. 60:1073, 1964.
4. Ellis, F. H., Jr., Callahan, J. A., McGoon, D. C., and Kirklin, J. W.: Results of open operation for acquired mitral-valve disease, N. Engl. J. Med. 272:869, 1965.
5. Hoeksema, T. D., Wallace, R. B., and Kirklin, J. W.: Closed mitral commissurotomy. Recent results in 291 cases, Am. J. Cardiol. 17:825, 1966.
6. Dahl, J. C., Winchell, P., and Borden, C. W.: Mitral stenosis. A long-term postoperative follow-up, Arch. Intern. Med. 119:92, 1967.
7. Glenn, W. W., Goodyear, A. V., Stansel, H. C., Jr., Calabrese, C., and Hume, H.: Mitral valvulotomy. II. Operative results after closed valvulotomy: A report of 500 cases, Am. J. Surg. 117:493, 1969.
8. Higgs, L. M., Glancy, D. L., O'Brien, K. P., Epstein, S. E., and Morrow, A. G.: Mitral restenosis: An uncommon cause of recurrent symptoms following mitral commissurotomy, Am. J. Cardiol. 26:34, 1970.
9. Keith, T. A., and Fowler, N. O.: Closed mitral commissurotomy. Complications and their effect on survival, Chest 61:24, 1972.
10. Nanda, N. C., Gramiak, R., Shah, P. M., and DeWeese, J. A.: Mitral commissurotomy versus replacement. Preoperative evaluation by echocardiography, Circulation 51:263, 1975.
11. Fraser, K., and Sugden, B. A.: Second closed mitral valvotomy for recurrent mitral stenosis, Thorax 32:759, 1977.
12. Spencer, F. C.: A plea for early, open mitral commissurotomy, Am. Heart J. 95:668, 1978.

Mitral Valve Stenosis Produced by or Worsened by Active Bacterial Endocarditis*

Bruce F. Waller, M.D., F.C.C.P.; Bruce M. McManus, M.D.; and William C. Roberts, M.D., F.C.C.P.

Regurgitation is the usual complication of active infective endocarditis involving a cardiac valve. The *development* of valve stenosis entirely from infective endocarditis, of course, is extremely rare and *worsening* of previously existing valve stenosis by infective endocarditis rarely has been documented. In this report we describe one patient who appeared to have mitral stenosis purely on the basis of a large vegetation filling much of the previously normal mitral orifice and another

*From the Pathology Branch, National Heart, Lung, and Blood Institute, National Institutes of Health, Bethesda. *Reprint requests: Dr. Roberts, Bldg 10A, Rm 3E30, National Heart, Lung and Blood Institute, Bethesda 20205*

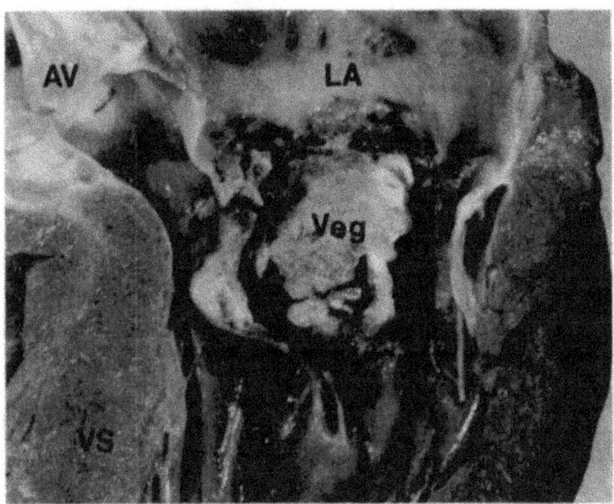

FIGURE 1 (Patient 1). Long axis view of heart showing a large vegetation (veg) in the mitral valve orifice of an otherwise normal mitral valve. AV = aortic valve, LA = left atrium, LV = left ventricle, VS = ventricular septum. (Photograph by M.M.M. Moore.)

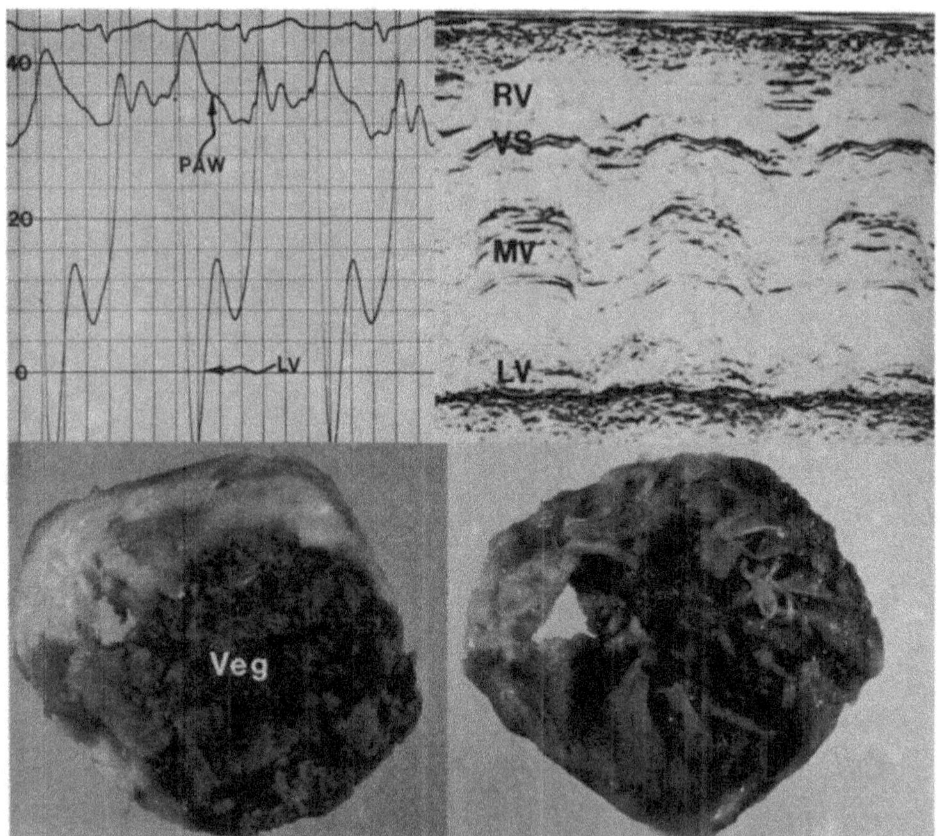

FIGURE 2 (Patient 2). *(Upper left):* Pressure tracing between pulmonary arterial wedge (PAW) position and left ventricle (LV) obtained one week before valve replacement showing a large diastolic gradient. *(Upper right):* M-mode echocardiogram typical of mitral stenosis. Excised mitral valve as seen from left atrium *(lower left)* and from left ventricle *(lower right).* Veg = vegetation. *(Photograph by M.M.M. Moore.)*

patient in whom active infection clearly worsened pre-existing mitral stenosis.

CASE REPORTS

The infecting bacterium in both patients was *Staphylococcus aureus.* Patient 1, a 71-year-old man, initially developed a murmur (grade 3/6) consistent with mitral regurgitation during his last two months of life while febrile (Fig 1). He died from intracerebral bleeding. Patient 2, a 37-year-old man who had had acute rheumatic fever as a child and a grade 1/6 apical diastolic rumble with a loud opening snap for at least three years, increased the intensity of the rumble to grade 3/6 and lost the opening snap when evidence of active infective endocarditis appeared. Cardiac catheterization during the infection disclosed a mean diastolic gradient of 26 mm Hg between pulmonary artery wedge position and left ventricle. The mitral valve was successfully replaced (Fig 2).

COMMENTS

Although hemodynamic confirmation is lacking, the finding of a large vegetation filling the mitral orifice of an otherwise normal valve in patient 1 strongly suggests that mitral stenosis can be produced by active infective endocarditis alone. Roberts and associates[1] previously reported the occurrence of mitral stenosis from infective endocarditis alone due to group B hemolytic Streptococcus in a 21-year-old woman at necropsy, and Davies and associates[2] later described a 38-year-old man in whom both the mitral and aortic orifices at operation appeared to have been obstructed by vegetations alone (group C hemolytic Streptococcus).

The occurrence of active infective endocarditis on a previously stenotic mitral valve, of course, may worsen the degree of stenosis although the degree of worsening has never been documented hemodynamically. In our patient 2 and in three previously reported patients,[3-5] the preexisting mitral stenosis was clearly worsened by the presence of vegetations. Of these four patients, the infecting bacterium in three was *Staphylococcus aureus,* and in one,[5] the blood cultures and cultures of the operatively-excised vegetations were negative. The excised mitral valves in the three previously reported patients were similar in appearance to that in our patient 2.

Thus, active infective endocarditis can by itself *produce* mitral stenosis, and active infective endocarditis may *worsen* preexisting mitral stenosis.

REFERENCES

1 Roberts WC, Evy GA, Glancy DL, Marcus FI. Valvular stenosis produced by active infective endocarditis. Circulation 1967; 36:449-51
2 Davies MK, Ireland MA, Clarke DB. Infective endocarditis from group C streptococci causing stenosis of both the aortic and mitral valves. Thorax 1981; 36:69-71

3 Reeve R, Reeve FJS, Matula G, Lawson W. Mitral obstruction by vegetations of staphylococcal endocarditis. JAMA 1974; 228:75

4 Matula G, Karpman LS, Frank S, Stinson EB. Mitral obstruction from Staphylococcal endocarditis, corrected surgically. JAMA 1975; 233:58-59

5 Copeland JG, Salomon NW, Stinson EB, Popp RL, Shumway NE. Acute mitral valvular obstruction from infective endocarditis. Echocardiographic diagnosis and report of the second successfully treated case. J Thorac Cardiovasc Surg 1979; 78:128-30

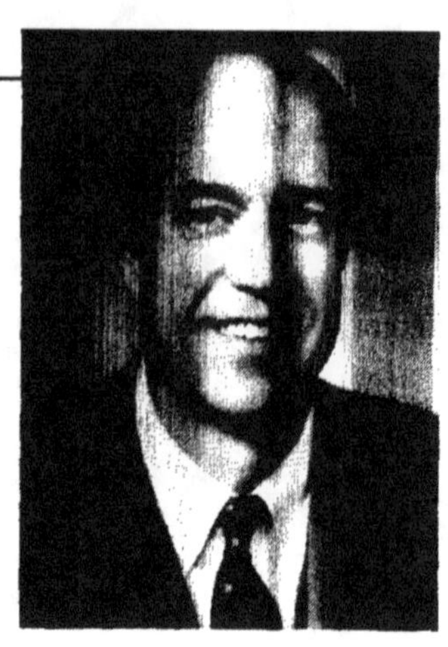

Mitral Commissurotomy—Still a Good Operation

Recently, I examined an operatively excised, severely stenotic mitral valve that was free of calcific deposits (by radiography of the excised valve) and of associated mitral regurgitation (by left ventricular angiography). The patient had no evidence of dysfunction of either the tricuspid or aortic valves. I asked the surgeon who had performed the mitral valve replacement (MVR) why that procedure was performed rather than mitral valve commissurotomy (MVC). I was surprised to hear that he "rarely did MVC anymore" and that he had "more confidence in MVR than in MVC." He had used a mechanical prosthesis for the MVR, which necessitated anticoagulant therapy for the rest of this 36-year-old woman's life. When I mentioned that chronic anticoagulant therapy would not have been necessary had MVC been performed, he responded that "MVR was still worth the difference." I disagree, and so does Bonchek[1] in the editorial in this issue.

In 1978, Lachman and I[2] radiographed 164 operatively excised stenotic mitral valves and quantitated the amount of calcific deposits in them. Of the 164 valves, 14 had absent and 43 minimal calcific deposits on x-ray examination of the excised valve. Of the 57 patients with absent or minimal calcific deposits, 37 had moderate to severe mitral regurgitation, and therefore, each clearly warranted MVR. The remaining 20 had absent or minimal calcific deposits and absent or minimal mitral regurgitation as determined by left ventricular angiography; nevertheless, MVR had been performed. We analyzed retrospectively those 20 patients to examine if MVR was preferable to MVC.[3]

To answer this question unequivocally, the stenotic mitral valves in patients who had only commissurotomy would have to be studied morphologically and radiographically in the same manner as those that were excised and replaced. Obviously, the nonexcised valve cannot be examined in the same manner as the excised valve.

Nevertheless, the ideal valve for MVC in the past has been considered to be the stenotic one that is free of calcific deposits, free of significant mitral regurgitation, and mobile. The excised mitral valves in the 20 patients whom we[3] analyzed were free of calcific deposits by preoperative examination (or nearly so by radiography of the excised valve, a far more sensitive technique than x-ray or fluoroscopy through the chest wall), and none had significant regurgitation by left ventricular angiography. The degree of mobility was infrequently described in the operative note. All 20 patients analyzed would probably have been acceptable candidates for MVC in the pre–valve replacement era. Why, then, might valve replacement be performed with its prosthetic- or bioprosthetic-related complications rather than MVC in this circumstance?

Of the 20 patients studied by Lachman and me,[3] several reasons appeared to account for MVR rather than MVC: (1) *Another cardiac valve was also replaced* (13 patients). Therefore, if the patient is required to have anticoagulant therapy for a prosthesis in the tricuspid or aortic valve position, MVR may be the more reasonable procedure and will avoid the risk of significant regurgitation or incomplete relief of the stenosis by MVC. (2) *Cardiopulmonary bypass was used* (all 20 patients). This procedure obviously allows visual inspection of the valve, something not possible when MVC is done as a "closed" procedure. I suspect that the visually inspected stenotic mitral valve is more frightening to the observer than is the palpated stenotic valve. Thus, visual inspection alone, particularly when valve replacement is a reasonable and uncriticized option, may push the surgeon toward replacement rather than simple commissurotomy in some patients. (3) *Some surgeons had relatively little experience with MVC* (17 patients). Of the 20 patients we analyzed, 17 were operated on by surgeons <40 years old when the operation was done. As pointed out by Bonchek,[1] younger surgeons have had much less experience with MVC than with MVR. (4) *Dissatisfaction with attempted MVC* (3 patients). (5) *Previous MVC had been performed* (11 patients). Although there is disagreement on this point, a mitral valve that has had a commissurotomy and later becomes severely stenotic can nevertheless have another MVC as long as calcific deposits are absent and regurgitation is absent or minimal. (6) *Incorrect identification of mitral calcific deposits* (2 patients). A calcific deposit was described in the mitral leaflets at operation, but x-ray of the excised valve showed that it was devoid of calcium.

Each of these 6 factors contributed in ≥ 1 of the 20 patients analyzed to the final operative decision of MVC rather than MVR. Even though MVC has been performed for >30 years, the mere alternative of MVR appears to have somewhat altered the definition of the mitral valve previously considered ideal for MVC. We need to return to the earlier definition of the ideal mitral valve suitable for MVC.

References

1. **Bonchek LI.** Current status of mitral commissurotomy: indications, techniques and results. Am J Cardiol 1983;52:411–414.
2. **Lachman AS, Roberts WC.** Calcific deposits in stenotic mitral valves. Extent and relationship to age, sex, degree of stenosis, cardiac rhythm, previous commissurotomy and left atrial body thrombus from study of 164 operatively-excised valves. Circulation 1978;57:808–815.
3. **Roberts WC, Lachman AS.** Mitral valve *commissurotomy* versus *replacement*. Considerations based on examination of operatively excised stenotic mitral valves. Am Heart J 1979;98:56–62.

William C. Roberts, MD
Editor-in-Chief

Relation of Level of Total Serum Cholesterol to Amount of Calcific Deposits in Operatively Excised Stenotic Mitral Valves: Analysis of 155 Cases

PAUL J. DAY* and WILLIAM C. ROBERTS, MD

This report analyzes 155 patients with rheumatic mitral stenosis in whom the operatively excised mitral valve was x-rayed to determine the presence of and extent of calcific deposits and the preoperative level of total serum cholesterol (TC). The amount of mitral calcium was graded 0 to 4+ and the average TC for each of the 5 groups was: 0 deposits—21 patients (14%) (TC = 188 mg/dl); 1+—50 patients (32%) (TC = 196 mg/dl); 2+—22 patients (14%) (TC = 198 mg/dl); 3+—37 patients (24%) (TC = 205 mg/dl), and 4+—25 patients (16%) (TC = 184 mg/dl). These average values of TC and the mean ages of the patients in each of the 5 groups of mitral calcium were not significantly different.

(Am J Cardiol 1984;53:157–159)

Mitral stenosis (MS) has been observed in persons residing in every continent and probably in every country on earth. In persons with MS living in Western countries, calcific deposits are usually found in stenotic mitral valves, and often, these deposits are quite heavy. In persons with MS living in undeveloped countries, in contrast, calcific deposits are usually not found in stenotic mitral valves and, when present, they are usually small. A major measurable difference between persons residing in developed Western countries and those residing in undeveloped countries is the serum total cholesterol (TC) level. We theorized that persons with calcific deposits, and particularly those with heavy deposits in stenotic mitral valves, would have higher TC levels than persons with MS and absent or small calcific deposits. To try to substantiate this thesis, we sought TC levels in a group of patients in whom we had x-rayed the operative excised stenotic mitral valve.

Methods

Each patient included in this study had undergone mitral valve replacement for MS with or without associated mitral regurgitation at the National Heart, Lung, and Blood Institute from 1963 through June 1983. Of approximately 400 mitral valve replacements for MS during this period, 194 operatively excised stenotic mitral valves had been x-rayed via a Field-Emission-Faxitron x-ray unit at 35 kVP. The x-ray beam was directed more or less perpendicular to the valve orifice. The presence of and the amount of calcium was determined by examination of the single radiograph of each excised mitral valve. The amount of calcium in each valve was graded by the percent of leaflet area occupied by calcium as follows: 0, no calcium; 1+, ≤25%; 2+, 26 to 50%; 3+, 51 to 75%; and 4+, 76 to 100%. The medical records in each of the 194 patients were reviewed to confirm the presence of a mean diastolic pressure gradient ≥5 mm Hg between pulmonary arterial wedge position (or left atrium) and left ventricle and to determine if a serum TC test had been performed in the 30 days preceding mitral valve replacement. Of the 194 patients with x-rays of the operatively excised mitral valve, all had hemodynamic evidence of MS as determined by cardiac catheterization before valve replacement, and 155 patients had TC determinations at some time during the 4 weeks before mitral valve replacement. These 155 patients constitute the study group for this report. Of the 155 patients, 118 had been included in an earlier analysis correlating the extent of calcific deposits in stenotic mitral valves to age, sex, degree of stenosis, cardiac rhythm, previous mitral commissurotomy and left atrial body thrombus.[1] The remaining 37 patients were studied since 1977. Of the 155 patients, 106 were women, aged 30 to 72 years (mean 53), and 49 were men, aged 28 to 74 years (mean 50). The mean diastolic pressure gradients from pulmonary arterial wedge position (or left atrium) to left ventricle in the 155 patients ranged from 5 to 30 mm Hg (mean 14).

Results

The amount of calcium present as determined from radiographs of the operatively excised mitral valves was as follows: 0—21 patients (14%); 1+—50 patients (32%); 2+—22 patients (14%); 3+—37 patients (24%); and

From the Pathology Branch, National Heart, Lung, and Blood Institute, National Institutes of Health, Bethesda, Maryland. Manuscript received and accepted August 15, 1983.

* Student, Saint Mary's College, Saint Mary's City, Maryland 20686.

Address for reprints: William C. Roberts, MD, Building 10A, Room 3E-30, National Institutes of Health, Bethesda, Maryland 20205.

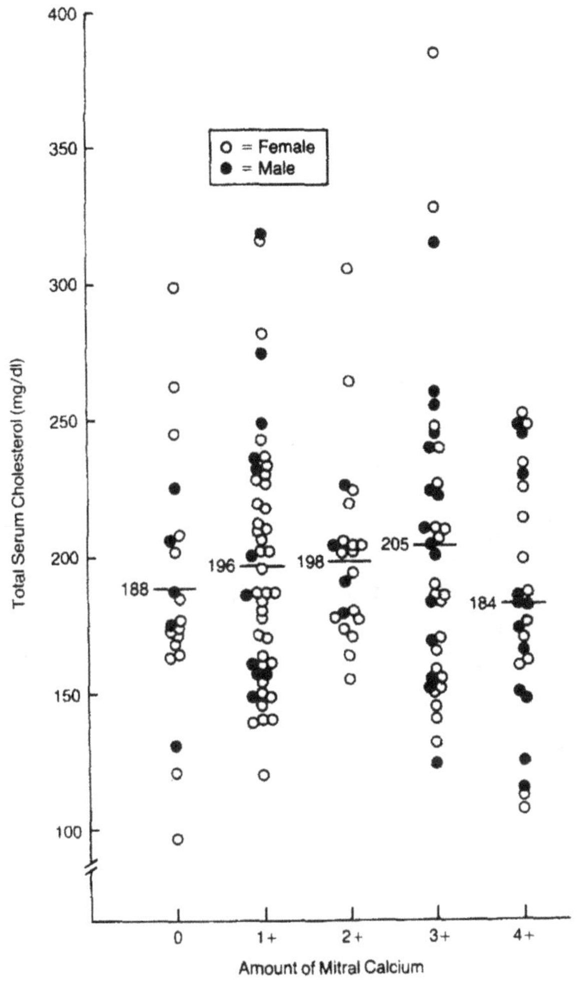

FIGURE 1. Relation of total serum cholesterol level to the amount of calcific deposits in the stenotic mitral valves of the 155 patients.

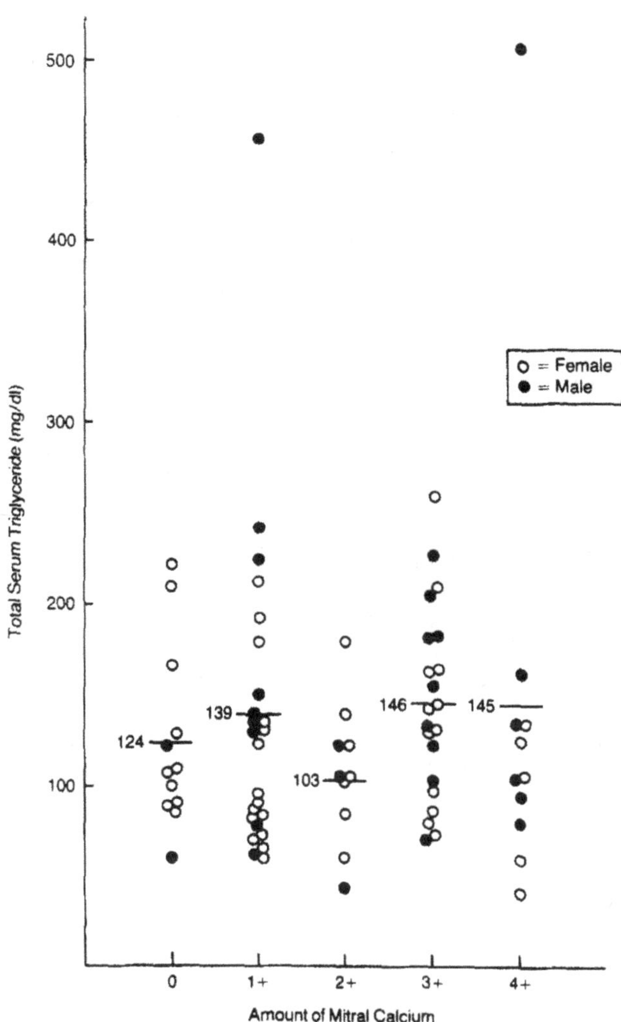

FIGURE 2. Relation of total serum triglyceride level to the amount of calcific deposits in the stenotic mitral valves in 77 of the 155 patients.

4+—25 patients (16%). The serum TC values in the 155 patients ranged from 107 to 385 mg/dl (mean 196); in the 106 women, the mean TC was 194 mg/dl and in the 49 men, 199 mg/dl. The TC values for each patient in each of the 5 categories of mitral calcific deposits are summarized in Figure 1. The means of the TC levels for each of the 5 categories of mitral calcific deposits were similar: in the 21 patients with no mitral calcific deposits, the TC averaged 188 mg/dl; for the 50 patients with 1+ mitral calcium, 196 mg/dl; for the 22 patients with 2+ calcium, 198 mg/dl; for the 37 patients with 3+ calcium, 205 mg/dl, and for the 25 patients with 4+ calcium, 184 mg/dl. These values were similar in both women and men (Fig. 1) in each of the 5 categories of mitral calcific deposits. The mean age of the patients in each of the 5 categories of mitral calcific deposits also was similar.

Fasting serum triglyceride levels in the 1 month preceding mitral valve replacement were available in 77 of the 155 patients, and the individual values relative to the amount of mitral calcium are summarized in Figure 2. No significant differences in the levels occurred in the 5 groups of mitral calcium.

Discussion

The above data indicate that the level of serum TC among our 155 adult patients with operatively excised stenotic mitral valves did not correlate with the amount of calcific deposits in the valve leaflets. Before dismissing any connection between the TC level and the amount of mitral calcium, however, it may be important to note that 89% of the patients (138 of 155) had TC levels >150 mg/dl, a level considered the lower range of normal in many medical centers in the United States. However, we consider this level the upper limit of normal because of the rarity of symptomatic atherosclerosis in persons with TC values below this level. Thus, we had only 17 patients with "normal" serum TC levels to compare with the 138 with elevated levels. Our 17 patients with TC levels ≤150 mg/dl, however, were fairly equally distributed among the 5 groups of patients with varying degrees of mitral calcium (Fig. 1).

No previous studies have described serum TC levels in patients with MS and no studies have described as much calcium in stenotic mitral valves as has our present and previous study.[1] Radiography of the operatively excised valve, however, is a far more sensitive means of determining the amount of calcium in a valve than is preoperative routine radiography, fluoroscopy or manual palpation at operation. Since other studies have not provided TC levels or data from radiographs of operatively excised valves, we cannot compare our present data to any other study.

Although several previous studies from Africa, Asia and Europe have described the amount of calcium in stenotic mitral valves as determined by manual palpation at the time of mitral commissurotomy, the patients were much younger than those of our study.[2-8] Stephen[7] in Sri Lanka performed mitral valve commissurotomy on 1,016 patients aged 6 to 63 years (mean 27), and 850 (84%) had no mitral calcific deposits, 123 (12%) had mild and only 43 (4%) had moderate to severe deposits. Nazarian and Aryanpur[6] in Iran described 62 patients aged 10 to 49 years at mitral valve replacement, and 37 (60%) had no palpable mitral calcium, 16 (26%) had mild deposits and 9 (14%) had moderate or heavy deposits. It is likely that most of the patients included in these 2 studies had total serum cholesterol levels ≤150 mg/dl. In contrast, Goodwin et al[2] in England described findings in 75 patients aged 17 to 58 years, and at mitral commissurotomy 47 (63%) had no mitral calcium, 22 (29%) had mild deposits and 6 (8%) had moderate or heavy deposits. It is likely that most of the latter 75 patients had serum TC levels >150 mg/dl, but again, the patients with the severe degrees of mitral calcium likely would be eliminated from the group of patients having mitral commissurotomy.

In conclusion, why some patients with MS have heavy calcific deposits in their stenotic valves and others have none or minimal deposits is not known. Age and sex, as determined earlier,[1] play a role, but other as yet unknown factors may play a larger role.

References

1. **Lachman AS, Roberts WC.** Calcific deposits in stenotic mitral valves. Extent and relation to age, sex, degree of stenosis, cardiac rhythm, previous commissurotomy and left atrial body thrombus from study of 164 operatively-excised valves. Circulation 1978;57:808–815.
2. **Goodwin JF, Hunter JD, Cleland WP, Davies LG, Steiner RE.** Mitral valve disease and mitral valvotomy. Br Med J 1955;2:573–585.
3. **Chesler E, Levin S, Du Plessis L, Freiman I, Rosers M, Joffe N.** The pattern of rheumatic heart disease in the urbanized Bantu of Johannesburg. S Afr Med J 1966;40:899–904.
4. **Knight EO, Kamdar HH, Chukwuemeka A.** Juvenile mitral stenosis in Kenya. East Afr Med J 1973;50:476–479.
5. **Adebonojo SA, Adebo O, Osinowo O.** Results of closed mitral commissurotomy for mitral stenosis at Ibadan. East Afr Med J 1979;56:485–489.
6. **Nazarian IH, Aryanpur I.** Pathology of chronic rheumatic mitral valvulitis in Iran and its surgical implications. Jpn Heart J 1978;19:1–11.
7. **Stephen SJ.** Mitral stenosis in Sri Lanka. Ceylon Med J 1979;24:13–20.
8. **Colman T, de Ubago JLM, Figueroa A, Pomar JL, Gallo I, Mortera C, Pajarón A, Durán CM.** Coronary arteriography and atrial thrombosis in mitral valve disease. Am J Cardiol 1981;47:973–977.

Amounts of Coronary Arterial Narrowing by Atherosclerotic Plaques in Clinically Isolated Mitral Valve Stenosis: Analysis of 76 Necropsy Patients Older Than 30 Years

RONALD N. REIS* and WILLIAM C. ROBERTS, MD

Although several studies have described the status of the coronary arteries by angiography in patients with mitral stenosis (MS), few necropsy studies of the coronary arteries in these patients are available. The present report describes in detail the amounts of narrowing by atherosclerotic plaque of the 4 major epicardial coronary arteries in 76 necropsy patients, aged 31 to 79 years (mean 53) with clinically isolated MS (with or without associated mitral regurgitation but without aortic valve dysfunction). Of the 76 patients, $\geq$1 major coronary artery was narrowed >75% in cross-sectional area (XSA) in 38 (50%) and in 10 of the 38 patients $\geq$1 major coronary artery was totally occluded or nearly so (>95% XSA narrowing). A higher percent of the 29 men had significant (>75% XSA) coronary narrowing than did the 47 women (62 vs 44%) and the men had more major coronary arteries significantly narrowed compared with the women (31 of 116 arteries [27%] vs 33 of 188 arteries [18%]).

The 4 major coronary arteries in the 76 patients were divided into 5-mm segments and examined histologically: of the 3,124 segments (41 per patient), 620 segments (20%) were narrowed 0 to 25% in XSA, 1,826 (58%) were narrowed 26 to 50%, 470 (15%) were narrowed 51 to 75%, 188 (6%) were narrowed 76 to 95%, and 20 segments (1%) were narrowed 96 to 100% in XSA. The percent of segments narrowed >75% in XSA was 9% in the men and 5% in the women. The percent of segments narrowed >75% in XSA was highly variable in the 38 patients with significant narrowing, ranging from 2 to 59% (mean 13%). Grossly visible left ventricular scars were present in 11 patients and in each they involved the posterior (inferior) wall; 8 of the 11 patients had significant coronary narrowing and 3 did not. Angina pectoris was present in 13 patients, 8 (62%) had significant coronary narrowing and 5 (38%) did not.

(Am J Cardiol 1986;57:1117–1123)

Although several reports have described coronary angiographic findings in patients with mitral stenosis (MS), few reports have described the frequency of and extent of coronary arterial narrowing at necropsy in patients with MS. In this report we describe the amounts of narrowing by atherosclerotic plaques observed at necropsy in the 4 major epicardial coronary arteries in 76 patients older than 30 years with clinically isolated MS with or without associated mitral regurgitation.

Methods

Patients classified as clinically isolated MS in the files of the Pathology Branch, National Heart, Lung, and Blood Institute (NHLBI), were reviewed and 76 patients fulfilled the following 4 criteria: (1) age >30 years at death; (2) presence of MS clinically and confirmation of MS at operation or at necropsy; (3) absence of clinical evidence of aortic valve dysfunction; (4) availability of the 4 major epicardial coronary arteries so that they could be examined in their entirety as discussed below. The hearts were received from 14 different medical centers: NHLBI = 39; Georgetown

*Sophomore Student, Albany Medical College, Albany, New York. From the Pathology Branch, National Heart, Lung, and Blood Institute, National Institutes of Health, Bethesda, Maryland. Manuscript received October 30, 1985, accepted December 6, 1985.

Address for reprints: William C. Roberts, MD, Building 10A, Room 3E-30, National Institutes of Health, Bethesda, Maryland 20205.

TABLE I   Clinical and Cardiac Morphologic Observations in the 47 Women with Mitral Stenosis

Pt	Age (yrs)	AP	AMI	Pressures (mm Hg)			LV Cine	Degree of MR (0–3+)	MVC	MVR	HW (g)	LA Clot	LV Scar	Major CAs >75% ↓ in XSA	5-mm CA Segs	5-mm Segments Narrowed in XSA (%)					Total	Mean
				LA	LV	LA-LV mdg										0–25	26–50	51–75	76–95	96–100		
1	31	0	0	—*(w)	—	—*	0	—	+	0	450	0	0	1	53	12	39	1	1	0	97	1.8
2	31	0	0	—*	—	—*	+	0	+	0	540	0	0	0	42	11	31	0	0	0	73	1.7
3	31	0	0	—*	—	—*	0	—	0	84 mos	520	0	0	0	33	17	16	0	0	0	49	1.5
4	32	0	0	15	96/6	5	+	0	+	0	560	+	0	0	26	7	17	2	0	0	47	1.8
5	33	0	0	21	106/3	13	+	1+	+	0	550	+	0	1	44	2	38	3	1	0	91	2.1
6	35	0	0	—(w)*	—	—*	0	—	0	2 mos	780	0	0	0	40	25	15	0	0	0	55	1.4
7	39	0	0	—*	—	—*	0	—	+	12 mos	380	0	0	0	38	9	25	4	0	0	71	1.9
8	40	0	0	35(w)	120/30	28	+	0	0	12 days	440	0	0	0	43	9	27	7	0	0	84	2.0
9	41	0	0	24	110/13	10	+	0	+	0	360	0	+	3	35	9	6	4	14	2	97	2.8
10	41	0	0	19	108/7	10	+	0	+	5 days	370	0	+	1	27	4	10	12	0	1	64	2.4
11	41	0	0	—*(w)	—	—*	+	1+	+	0	450	+(LAA)	0	0	54	2	48	4	0	0	110	2.0
12	42	0	0	30(w)	125/10	24	+	3+	0	5 days	460	0	0	0	45	9	35	1	0	0	82	1.8
13	43	0	0	14(w)	150/12	5	+	3+	+	24 mos	540	0	0	0	43	33	10	0	0	0	53	1.2
14	44	0	0	20	95/6	20	+	3+	+	4 days	450	0	0	0	42	9	33	0	0	0	75	1.8
15	44	0	0	24(w)	95/20	14	0	—	+	1 day	480	0	0	1	45	6	10	24	5	0	118	2.6
16	47	+	0	—	—	—	0	—	0	0	430	0	0	1	42	2	25	8	7	0	104	2.5
17	47	0	0	18(w)	105/2	22	+	1+	0	22 days	380	0	0	0	35	3	27	5	0	0	72	2.1
18	48	0	+(po)	23	84/7	9	+	0	+	62 mos	510	0	0	0	38	14	24	0	0	0	62	1.6
19	48	+	0	—	—	—	0	—	0	0	370	0	0	0	43	23	12	8	0	0	71	1.7
20	49	+	0	—	—	—	0	—	+	0	525	0	0	3	36	0	17	11	8	0	99	2.8
21	50	+	0	18	112/7	12	+	0	+	0	465	+	0	0	38	3	33	2	0	0	75	2.0
22	52	0	0	30(w)	120/20	21	+	2+	0	0	645	+	+	2	50	16	17	11	6	0	107	2.1
23	54	+	0	19	136/10	12	+	3+	0	24 days	630	0	0	1	34	6	19	7	1	1	73	2.1
24	55	0	0	31(w)	137/12	26	+	2+	0	1 mo	420	0	0	1	37	2	30	4	1	0	78	2.1
25	56	+	0	14(w)	108/7	13	+	2+	+	OR	500	0	+	3	57	14	13	13	15	2	147	2.6
26	59	+	0	18(w)	130/16	7	+	3+	0	77 mos	540	0	0	0	47	15	28	4	0	0	83	1.8
27	59	+	0	20(w)	150/12	11	+	0	+	7 yrs	550	0	0	0	29	6	23	0	0	0	52	1.8
28	59	0	0	—*	—	10	+	1+	0	7 yrs	—	0	0	0	33	13	20	0	0	0	53	1.6
29	60	+	0	40(w)	160/15	22	+	1+	0	12 days	470	0	0	1	43	10	29	3	1	0	81	1.9
30	61	0	0	26(w)	105/8	10	+	2+	0	6 days	540	0	0	0	44	11	33	0	0	0	77	1.8
31	62	0	0	14(w)	120/8	11	0	—	0	5 mos	380	0	0	2	42	8	10	22	2	0	102	2.4
32	62	0	0	15(w)	120/5	16	+	1+	0	36 hrs	520	0	0	0	42	10	32	0	0	0	74	1.8
33	62	0	0	—*	140/6	6	+	3+	0	<1 day	660	0	0	1	25	12	7	5	1	0	45	1.3
34	62	0	0	13(w)	118/15	6	+	3+	0	3 hrs	500	0	0	0	46	21	23	2	0	0	73	1.6
35	64	0	0	25(w)	135/8	18	+	0	+	0	410	0	0	0	41	5	36	0	0	0	77	1.9
36	64	0	0	16(w)	—	10	+	0	+	0	420	0	0	2	37	3	20	7	7	0	92	2.5
37	65	0	0	—	—	—*	0	—	0	0	370	0	0	1	33	15	15	2	1	0	55	1.7
38	65	0	0	25	120/15	9	+	3+	0	6 days	640	0	0	0	38	20	18	0	0	0	56	1.5
39	65	0	0	—*	—	—*	0	—	0	OR	440	0	0	0	32	8	21	3	0	0	59	1.8
40	66	0	0	29(w)	110/16	13	+	3+	0	4 mos	560	0	0	1	48	7	32	7	2	0	100	2.1
41	68	0	0	—*	—	—*	0	—	0	13 yrs	545	0	0	3	52	3	20	17	11	1	142	2.7
42	69	0	0	30(w)	120/8	17	+	1+	+	0	380	+(LAA)	0	0	25	4	15	6	0	0	52	2.1
43	70	0	0	—	—	—	0	—	0	0	320	0	0	0	49	7	42	0	0	0	91	1.9
44	75	0	0	—	—	—	0	—	0	0	420	0	0	1	43	0	28	13	2	0	103	2.4
45	77	0	0	16(w)	100/14	12	+	0	0	2 mos	315	0	0	0	41	9	29	3	0	0	76	1.9
46	77	0	0	—*	—	—*	+	0	+	2 days	495	+	0	3	32	0	13	15	2	2	87	2.7
47	79	0	0	45(w)	155/15	20	+	0	+	0	625	+	0	0	42	10	24	8	0	0	82	2.0

* Known to be elevated but numbers not available. AMI = acute myocardial infarction; AP = angina pectoris; CA = coronary artery; HW = heart weight; LA = left atrium; LV = left ventricle; mdg = mean diastolic gradient; MR = mitral regurgitation; MVC = mitral valve commissurotomy; MVR = mitral valve replacement; OR = death in operating room; Segs = segments; w = pulmonary artery wedge pressure; XSA = cross-sectional area.

University Medical Center = 14; National Naval Medical Center = 8; District of Columbia Medical Examiners Office = 3; Suburban Hospital = 2; Franklin Square Hospital (Baltimore) = 2; and 1 came from each of 9 other medical centers. Of the 76 cases, in 3 (4%) necropsy had been performed in the 1950s, in 17 (22%) in the 1960s, in 21 (28%) in the 1970s, and in 35 (46%) in the 1980s.

In each of the 76 patients the clinical records were examined, the heart was reexamined, and the 4 major (right, left main, left anterior descending and left circumflex) epicardial coronary arteries were excised intact from the heart, decalcified if necessary, divided into 5-mm long segments, cut transversely to the long axis of the artery, labeled sequentially from the origin of the artery from either the aorta or left main coronary artery, processed in alcohols and xylene, embedded in paraffin, cut 6 μ thick, and at least 1 histologic section from each 5-mm segment was stained by the Movat method and examined.[1] The degree of cross-sectional area (XSA) narrowing by atherosclerotic plaques was determined by examining the Movat-stained sections, which clearly delineate the internal elastic membrane. The amount of XSA luminal narrowing was determined by magnifying each cross section of coronary artery 40 times via microscopy and estimating the degrees of luminal obliteration by visually dividing the XSA of the coronary artery into 4 quadrants, each comprising 25% of the total XSA luminal area. The degrees of XSA narrowing were categorized initially into 4 groups: 0 to 25, 26 to 50, 51 to 75 and 76 to 100%. All sections narrowed >75% were further classified into a group with narrowing 76 to 95% and into a group with narrowing 96 to 100% in XSA. Both the inter- and intraobserver error by this technique is <5%.[2]

The 76 patients ranged in age from 31 to 79 years (mean 53): 47 patients (62%) were women (mean age 54 years) (Table I) and 29 (38%) were men (mean age 51 years) (Table II). Ischemic-type chest pains occurred in 14 patients (18%): angina pectoris in 13 patients (17%) and clinical features diagnostic of acute myocardial infarction in 1 patient (1%). Of the 76 patients, left-sided cardiac catheterization was performed in 66 patients (87%); the catheterization data shown in Tables I and II are those recorded just before mitral valve replacement or if no valve replacement the data recorded at the last catheterization, usually many years after mitral commissurotomy if that procedure had been done. The mean diastolic gradient between left atrium or pulmonary arterial wedge position and left ventricle (52 patients) ranged from 5 to 28 mm Hg (average mean gradient 15 mm Hg). The degree of mitral regurgitation by left ventricular angiography (52 patients) was graded 0 (absent) (18 patients), 1+ (mild) (13 patients), 2+ (moderate) (8 patients) and 3+ (severe) (13 patients). Of the 76 patients, mitral valve commissurotomy had been performed in 32 patients (42%) and mitral valve replacement in 47. Of the 76 patients, 64 patients (84%) had either mitral valve commissurotomy (17 patients [27%]) or mitral valve replacement (32 patients [50%]) or both (15 patients [23%]). Of the 32 patients having commissurotomy, the commissurotomy had been performed >1 year before death in all

but 2 patients, who died just after the procedure. The replacement was performed within 30 days of death in 30 patients (64%), from 2 to 12 months of death in 6 patients (13%) and from 24 to 156 months (mean 95) before death in 11 patients (23%).

At necropsy, the hearts of the 47 women weighed 315 to 780 g (mean 485) (normal ≤350 g), and the hearts of the 29 men weighed 410 to 800 g (mean 559) (normal ≤400 g). Although functionally normal, each of the 3 aortic valve cusps were thickened in 17 patients: nos. 8, 11, 12, 26, 33, 38 and 46 in Table I and patients 1, 5 to 7, 11, 15, 20, 23, 25 and 27 in Table II.

A grossly visible left ventricular scar (healed myocardial infarction) was found at necropsy in 11 patients (14%): in 1 patient the scar was limited to the inner half of the left ventricular wall (endocardial) and in 10 patients the scar involved both inner and outer half of the left ventricular wall (transmural); in 9 patients the left ventricular scars were small and in 2 patients they were large (patients no. 9 and no. 17, Table II). The scars involved only the posterior (or inferior) left ventricular wall in 10 patients and both anterior and posterior walls in 1 patient (no. 17, Table II). Of the 11 patients with grossly visible left ventricular scars, 8 had narrowing by atherosclerotic plaque >75% in XSA of ≥1 of the 4 major epicardial coronary arteries and 3 did not.

Thrombi were present at operation or at necropsy in the left atrial cavity in 14 patients (18%). The thrombi were limited to the appendage in 3 patients and involved both left atrial appendage and body in 11 patients. Of the 14 patients with left atrial thrombi, 7 had narrowing >75% in XSA of ≥1 of the 4 major epicardial coronary arteries.

Only 2 patients (patient 25, Table I, and patient 4, Table II) had coronary artery bypass grafting. Both

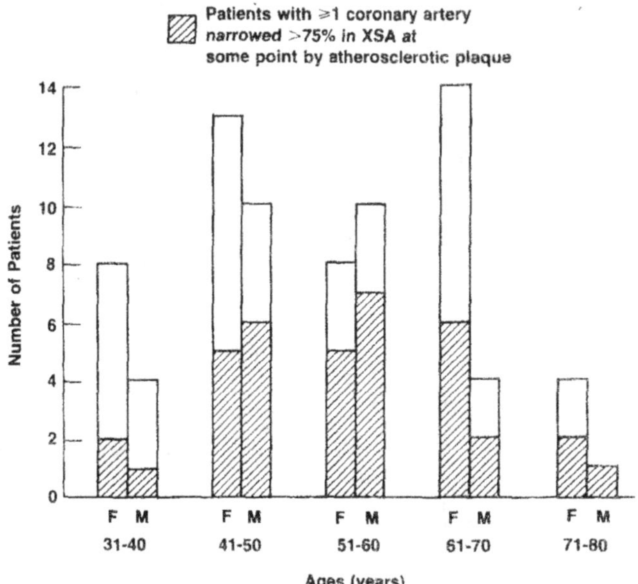

FIGURE 1. Number of necropsy patients by age decade and sex with clinically isolated mitral stenosis, with or without associated mitral regurgitation, in whom ≥1 major epicardial coronary artery was narrowed 76 to 100% in cross-sectional area at some point by atherosclerotic plaque.

TABLE II Clinical and Cardiac Morphologic Findings in the 29 Men with Mitral Stenosis

Pt	Age (yrs)	AP	AMI	Pressures (mm Hg) LA	LV	LA-LV mdg	LV Cine	Degree of MR (0–3+)	MVC	MVR	HW (g)	LA Clot	LV Scar	No. of 4 Major CAs >75% ↓ in XSA	No. of 5-mm CA Segs	No. of 5-mm Segments Narrowed in XSA (%) 0–25	26–50	51–75	76–95	96–100	Total	Mean
1	31	0	0	16	93/6	12	+	2+	+	5d	570	+(po)	0	0	29	7	22	0	0	0	51	1.8
2	38	0	0	16	85/2	16	+	2+	0	2d	445	0	+	0	39	9	26	4	0	0	73	1.9
3	40	0	0	24	110/12	13	+	3+	0	2d	680	0	0	0	44	14	27	3	0	0	77	1.8
4	40	+	+po	26(w)	104/4	20	+	0	0	10h	495	0	0	1	27	0	25	1	1	0	57	2.1
5	42	0	0	27	100/9	19	0	—	+	0	480	0	0	2	43	0	18	20	5	0	116	2.7
6	42	0	0	17	135/2	20	+	0	+	0	470	0	0	0	19	0	16	3	0	0	41	2.2
7	44	0	0	34	129/10	21	0	—	0	6d	530	+	0	1	35	5	24	5	1	0	72	2.1
8	45	0	0	24	105/9	16	+	1+	0	4d	—	+	0	2	49	19	21	7	2	0	90	1.8
9	47	0	0	37(w)	100/21	17	+	2+	0	13d	570	+(po)	+	1	55	13	11	19	11	1	140	2.6
10	47	+	0	—	—	—	0	—	+	0	530	0	0	1	43	3	29	10	1	0	95	2.2
11	49	+	0	34	165/13	14	0	0	+	29d	665	0	+	3	39	1	10	19	9	0	114	2.9
12	49	0	0	32	86/7	17	0	—	0	0	410	0	0	1	38	0	27	10	1	0	88	2.3
13	49	0	0	30	105/5	17	+	3+	+	6h	800	0	0	0	31	1	28	2	0	0	63	2.0
14	50	0	0	25	110/11	15	+	2+	+	135m	600	0	0	0	50	9	41	0	0	0	91	2.8
15	51	0	0	41	—	—	0	—	0	0	480	+	0	0	49	0	48	1	0	0	99	2.0
16	52	0	0	—*	—	—*	+	1+	0	10y	490	0	0	0	53	19	31	3	0	0	90	1.7
17	53	0	+	—	—	—	0	—	0	0	445	0	+†	3	64	0	11	15	30	8	219	3.4
18	53	0	0	—	—	—	0	—	0	0	420	0	0	1	43	1	35	6	1	0	93	2.2
19	53	0	0	—*(w)	—	11	+	1+	0	11d	520	0	+	0	33	0	32	1	0	0	67	2.0
20	53	0	0	—*(w)	—	14	+	1+	0	0	470	0	0	3	49	4	29	8	7	1	118	2.4
21	54	0	0	22(w)	100/12	14	+	3+	+	87m	940	0	+	1	37	0	19	15	2	1	95	2.6
22	54	0	0	—*	—	—*	+	0	+	0	480	0	0	2	32	2	21	5	4	0	75	2.3
23	54	0	0	—*	—	—*	+	0	+	OR	420	+	0	1	43	1	20	20	2	0	109	2.5
24	56	0	0	—*(w)	—	25	0	—	0	17d	580	0	0	1	35	8	23	3	1	0	67	1.9
25	62	0	0*	25	155/17	7	+	3+	0	5d	720	0	0	3	88	0	49	27	12	0	227	2.6
26	65	0	0	28(w)	100/0	10	+	1+	+	11y	760	+	0	0	44	1	43	0	0	0	87	2.0
27	66	+	0	—*	—	—*	0	—	+	0	600	0	+	0	60	47	12	1	0	0	74	1.2
28	66	0	0	—*(w)	—	10	+	1+	0	9m	620	0	0	1	29	10	15	0	4	0	56	1.9
29	75	0	0	39(w)	—	—*	0	—	0	0	410	+(LAA)	0	3	40	2	18	14	6	0	104	2.6

* Numbers not available but known to be increased.
† Also healing anterior wall myocardial infarct.
Abbreviations as in Table I.

patients also had mitral valve replacement; 1 died in the operating room and the other within 10 hours after operation.

Results

Of the 76 necropsy patients, 38 (50%) had ≥1 of their 4 major epicardial coronary arteries narrowed >75% in XSA by atherosclerotic plaques (Fig. 1): in 22 patients (29%), 1 of the 4 arteries was so narrowed; in 6 patients (8%), 2 such arteries, and in 10 patients (13%) 3 such arteries. Thus, in the 38 patients, 64 major coronary arteries were narrowed >75% in XSA, an average of 1.7 coronary arteries per patient; of the entire 76 patients, an average of 0.8 coronary arteries were so narrowed.

Of the 47 women, 20 (44%) had ≥1 of the 4 major coronary arteries narrowed >75% in XSA by plaque and of the 29 men, 18 (62%) had ≥1 major coronary artery so narrowed. Not only did a higher percent of the men have narrowing ≥1 major coronary artery >75% in XSA by plaque, but a higher percent of their 4 major coronary arteries were so narrowed. Of the 188 major epicardial coronary arteries examined in the 47 women, 33 (18%) were narrowed at some point >75% in XSA by plaque; of the 116 major coronary arteries examined in the 29 men, 31 (27%) were narrowed >75% in XSA by plaque. Of the 304 major coronary arteries examined in the 76 patients, 64 (21%) were narrowed at some point >75% in XSA by plaque. Of the 64 coronary arteries narrowed >75% in XSA at some point, the right coronary artery was so narrowed in 26 patients (41%), the anterior descending in 22 (34%), the left circumflex in 16 (25%) and the left main in none. Of the 38 patients with ≥1 coronary artery narrowed >75% in XSA by plaque, 8 (21%) had a grossly visible left ventricular scar. The other 3 patients with grossly visible left ventricular scars had insignificant coronary arterial narrowing.

A total of 3,124 five-millimeter segments of the 304 major epicardial coronary arteries in the 76 patients were examined (Fig. 2): 620 segments (20%) were narrowed 0 to 25% in XSA by atherosclerotic plaque; 1,826 segments (58%) were narrowed 26 to 50%; 470 segments (15%) were narrowed 51 to 75%; 188 segments (6%) were narrowed 76 to 95% and 20 segments (1%) were narrowed 96 to 100% in XSA. The percent of 5-mm segments narrowed >75% in XSA was nearly 2 times higher in the men than in the women: of the 1,240 five-millimeter segments examined in the 29 men, 111 (9%) were narrowed >75% in XSA and of the 1,884 segments examined in the 47 women, 97 (5%) were narrowed >75% in XSA.

Among the 38 patients in whom narrowing >75% in XSA was present in ≥1 major coronary artery, the number and percent of 5-mm segments narrowed to this extent varied greatly. Among the 38 patients with significant (>75% in XSA) coronary arterial narrowing, 1,604 five-millimeter segments were examined and of them 208 segments (13%) were narrowed >75% in XSA: of the 815 segments examined in the 20 women, 97 (12%) were narrowed >75%. Of the 38 patients, however, with narrowing >75% of ≥1 coronary artery, 13 patients (34%) had only a single 5-mm segment narrowed to this degree, 6 (16%) others had only 2 segments so narrowed, and 6 (16%) others had 3 to 5 segments so narrowed. Thus, 25 (66%) of the 38 patients had ≤5 coronary segments narrowed >75% in XSA, and only 6 patients (16%) had >10 segments severely narrowed. The percent of 5-mm segments narrowed >75% in XSA in the 38 patients ranged from 2 to 59% (mean 13%).

The number and percent of 5-mm coronary segments totally occluded or nearly so (>95% in XSA) also varied greatly. Only 10 of the 76 patients had any coronary segment narrowed to this degree and all but 1 of them also had ≥1 coronary segment also narrowed

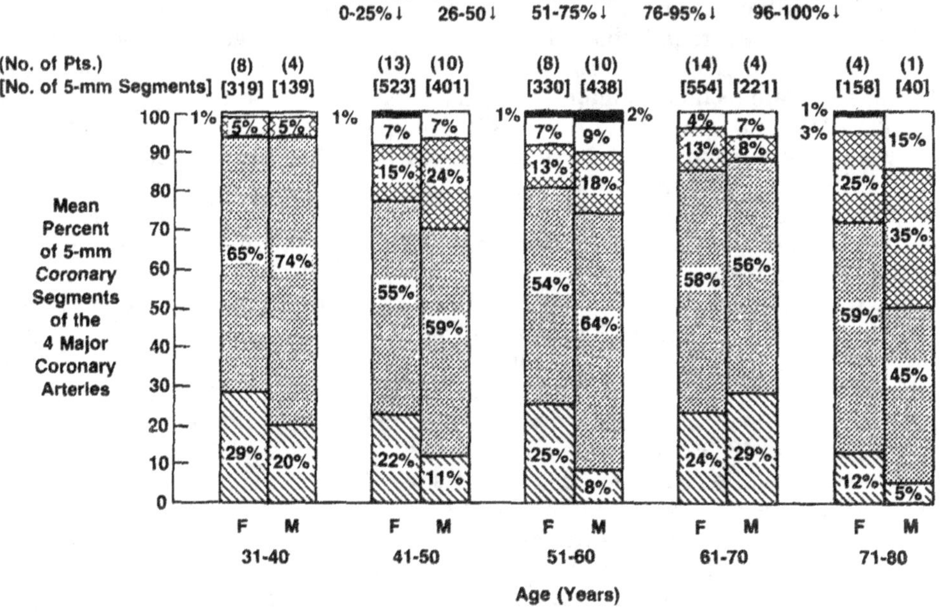

FIGURE 2. Number and percent of 3,124 five-millimeter segments of the 4 major epicardial coronary arteries narrowed to various degrees by atherosclerotic plaque in 76 patients (47 women, 29 men) aged 31 to 79 years with clinically isolated mitral stenosis with or without associated mitral regurgitation.

TABLE III Degrees of Coronary Arterial Narrowing By Angiogram During Life and at Necropsy in 13 Patients with Mitral Stenosis and Coronary Angiography

Table No.	Age (yr) & Sex	Maximal Narrowing by Angiogram (%DR)				Maximal Narrowing by Histology at Necropsy (%XSA)					
		R	LM	LAD	LC	R	LM	LAD	LC	AP	CABG
I	40F	0	0	0	0	51–75	51–75	51–75	26–50	0	0
I	54F	0	0	0	0	51–75	26–50	76–100	26–50	0	0
I	55F	25	0	25	0	51–75	26–50	76–100	26–50	0	0
I	56F	100	0	65	65	76–100	51–75	76–100	76–100	+	+
I	59F	0	0	0	0	51–75	0–25	26–50	26–50	0	+
I	62F	0	0	0	0	26–50	0–25	26–50	26–50	0	0
I	65F	0	0	0	0	26–50	26–50	26–50	26–50	0	0
I	69F	0	0	0	0	51–75	—	51–75	26–50	0	0
II	40M	0	0	50	95	51–75	—	26–50	76–100	+	+
II	52M	0	0	0	0	51–75	26–50	26–50	0–25	0	0
II	53M	0	0	0	0	26–50	26–50	26–50	51–75	0	0
II	54M	0	0	0	0	51–75	26–50	76–100	51–75	0	0
II	65M	0	0	0	0	26–50	26–50	26–50	26–50	0	0

AP = angina pectoris; CABG = coronary artery bypass grafting; DR = diameter reduction; LAD = left anterior descending coronary artery; LC = left circumflex coronary artery; LM = left main coronary artery; R = right coronary artery; XSA = cross-sectional area.

76 to 95% in XSA. Of these 10 patients, only 1 or 2 coronary segments were narrowed >95% in XSA in 9 patients; in the other patients, 8 of 38 segments (21%) were narrowed to this extent. Thus, of the 1,604 five-millimeter coronary segments narrowed >75% in XSA in the 38 patients, 20 segments (1%) were narrowed >95% in XSA.

A scoring system also was used to indicate the severity and extent of coronary arterial narrowing. Every 5-mm segment of coronary artery from each patient was assigned a score of 1 to 4 based on the amount of XSA narrowing by atherosclerotic plaque: 1 = 0 to 25% narrowing; 2 = 26 to 50%; 3 = 51 to 75% and 4 = 76 to 100%. A total score was determined for each patient and the mean score per segment was then calculated by dividing the total score per patient by the number of segments examined from that patient. The total score for the 3,124 five-millimeter coronary segments from the 76 patients was 6,514, indicating that the mean score for each 5-mm segment was 2.1. The latter number indicates that the amount of XSA narrowing for the 3,124 segments averaged about 40%.

Of the 10 patients with grossly visible left ventricular scars, 7 patients had ≥1 major coronary artery narrowed >75% and in 6 of the 7 patients ≥1 major coronary artery was narrowed >95% in XSA. Of the 496 five-millimeter coronary segments examined in these 10 patients, the total score was 1,197 for an average of 2.4 per segment, a number higher than that for the entire 76 patients.

Of the 13 patients with angina pectoris, 8 (62%) had narrowing >75% in XSA of ≥1 major epicardial coronary artery and 3 of the 13 patients (23%) also had grossly visible left ventricular scars. A total of 538 five-millimeter coronary segments were examined in these 13 patients and 46 (9%) of them were narrowed >75% in XSA. The total score in the 538 segments was 1,125, indicating a mean score of 2.1 per segment or approximately 40% XSA narrowing per segment.

Coronary angiography had been performed in life in 13 patients (Table III) and 2 patients (15%) had >50% diameter narrowing of ≥1 major epicardial coronary artery. At necropsy (within 2 months of angiography), 3 other patients—a total of 5—had narrowing >75% in XSA.

Discussion

This study demonstrates that 38 (50%) of our 76 necropsy patients over 30 years of age with clinically isolated MS (with or without associated mitral regurgitation but without aortic valve dysfunction) had narrowing of ≥1 major epicardial coronary artery between 76 and 95% in XSA by atherosclerotic plaque and that 10 of the 38 patients had XSA narrowing >95% in XSA by plaque. A higher percent of men than women had significant (>75% in XSA) narrowing of ≥1 major coronary artery (62% vs 44%). Moreover, the men had a higher number of major coronary arteries narrowed >75% in XSA than did the women (31 [27%] the 116 major coronary arteries in the 29 men vs 33 [18%] of the 188 major coronary arteries in the 47 women). Grossly visible left ventricular scars and/or angina pectoris were relatively infrequent in the patients with or without significant coronary narrowing. Of the 38 patients with narrowing >75% in XSA of ≥1 major coronary artery, only 8 (21%) had a grossly visible left ventricular scar and of the 38 without a major coronary artery narrowed >75% in XSA 3 (8%) had a grossly visible left ventricular scar. Of the 38 patients with significant coronary narrowing, 8 (21%) had angina pectoris and of the 38 patients in whom none of the major coronary arteries were narrowed >75% in XSA, 5 (13%) had had angina. Of the 64 coronary arteries narrowed >75% in XSA (average 1.7 per patient) in the 38 patients, the right one was narrowed most frequently (41% vs 34% for the left anterior descending and 25% for the left circumflex). The posterior (inferior) wall was the location of the grossly visible left ventricular scars in all 11 patients with scars.

Of the 3,124 five-millimeter segments of the 4 major epicardial coronary arteries examined in the 76 patients (mean 41 per patient), 188 segments (6%) were narrowed 76 to 95% in XSA and 20 segments (1%) were narrowed 96 to 100% in XSA. The percent of segments narrowed >75% in XSA was nearly twice as high in the men compared to the women. In the 38 patients in whom at least 1 segment was narrowed >75% in XSA, a total of 1,604 five-millimeter coronary segments were examined and 208 (13%) were narrowed >75% in XSA; the percent of segments narrowed >75% in XSA varied in these 38 patients from as few as 2% to as many as 59%. Of the 10 patients in whom at least 1 coronary segment was narrowed >95% in XSA, only 1 or 2 segments were narrowed to this degree in 9 patients.

Although one-half of the 76 patients had narrowing of >75% in XSA of at least 1 major coronary artery, the length of the narrowing, i.e., the number of 5-mm segments narrowed to this degree, was much less than in necropsy patients with fatal coronary heart disease studied in a similar fashion. Among 31 victims of sudden coronary death studied in this laboratory, 36% of the 5-mm segments of the 4 major coronary arteries were narrowed >75% in XSA by atherosclerotic plaque[3]; the percent in 27 victims of transmural acute myocardial infarction was 34%[4]; the percent in 22 patients with unstable angina pectoris was 48%,[5] and the percent in patients with healed myocardial infarction was 31%.[6–8]

The only other major necropsy study of the coronary arteries in patients with MS was by Tadavarthy et al.[9] These authors examined the major epicardial coronary arteries, primarily by gross inspection of cross sections of the arteries, of 60 patients, 47 women, aged "20s" to "70s" (mean "50s") with pure MS. Of the 60 patients, 21 (35%) had "significant" obstructive lesions in ≥1 major coronary artery: of the 47 women, 15 (32%) had ≥1 "severe" coronary narrowing and of the 13 men, 6 (46%) had ≥1 severe coronary narrowing. Of the 21 patients with significant coronary narrowing, 1 major artery was severely narrowed in 6 patients (29%), 2 arteries in 8 patients (38%), 3 arteries in 6 patients (14%) and 4 arteries in 1 patient (5%). As in the present study, the right coronary artery was more frequently severely narrowed than was the left anterior descending or the left circumflex.

Although morphologic studies of the coronary arteries in MS have been rare, several angiographic studies of the coronary arteries in patients with MS have been reported.[10–16] Befeler et al[10] performed coronary arteriography in 26 patients aged 32 to 69 years (mean 45) with isolated MS and found 5 patients (19%) to have >50% diameter reduction in ≥1 major coronary artery (complete obstruction in 4); 3 patients (12%) had clinical evidence of healed myocardial infarction, 2 with 100% obstruction and 1 with 50% obstruction of a coronary artery; and 3 (12%) patients had angina pectoris (1 also had a healed myocardial infarct) and all 3 had 100% obstruction of a coronary artery. Lacy et al[11] studied 67 patients (49 women) with "predominant" MS and by angiograms 13 (19%) had ≥1 coronary artery narrowed >50% in diameter: 3 arteries so narrowed in 1 patient, 2 arteries so narrowed in 6 patients,

and 1 artery so narrowed in 6 patients. Chun and associates[12] found angiographically significant (>50% diameter reduction) coronary narrowing in 16 (20%) of 82 patients (mean age 51 years, 47 women) with MS. Saltups[13] by angiography found ≥1 coronary arterial narrowing ≥50% in diameter in 7 (10%) of 68 patients with MS: angina was present in 4 and absent in 3 of the 7 patients with significant coronary narrowing; none of the 61 patients without significant coronary narrowing had angina. Ramsdale et al[14] found coronary arterial narrowing ≥50% diameter reduction in 24 (28%) of 86 patients with MS: of the 21 patients with angina pectoris, 13 had angiographically significant coronary narrowing and 8 did not. Czer and associates[15] found ≥50% diameter reduction of ≥1 major coronary artery by angiogram in 57 (29%) of 199 patients with MS in whom mitral valve replacement was performed. Mattina and colleagues[16] found ≥1 major coronary artery narrowed ≥70% in diameter in 27 (28%) of 96 patients aged 41 to 74 years (mean 60) (73 women) with severe MS; 21 (22%) of the 96 patients had angina pectoris and 10 of them had angiographically significant coronary narrowing and 11 did not.

References

1. Movat HZ. Demonstration of all connective tissue elements in a single section: pentachrome stains. Arch Pathol 1955;60:289–295.
2. Isner JM, Wu M, Renu V, Jones AA, Roberts WC. Comparison of degrees of coronary arterial luminal narrowing determined by visual inspection of histologic sections under magnification among three independent observers and comparison to that obtained by video planimetry. An analysis of 559 five-millimeter segments of 61 coronary arteries from eleven patients. Lab Invest 1980;42:566–570.
3. Roberts WC, Jones AA. Quantitation of coronary arterial narrowing at necropsy in sudden coronary death. Analysis of 31 patients and comparison with 25 control subjects. Am J Cardiol 1979;44:39–45.
4. Roberts WC, Jones AA. Quantification of coronary arterial narrowing at necropsy in acute transmural myocardial infarction: analysis and comparison of findings in 27 patients and 22 controls. Circulation 1980;61:786–790.
5. Roberts WC, Virmani R. Quantification of coronary arterial narrowing in clinically-isolated unstable angina pectoris. An analysis of 22 necropsy patients. Am J Med 1979;67:792–799.
6. Virmani R, Roberts WC. Quantification of coronary arterial narrowing and of left ventricular myocardial scarring in healed myocardial infarction with chronic eventually fatal, congestive cardiac failure. Am J Med 1980;68:831–838.
7. Cabin HS, Roberts WC. True left ventricular aneurysm and healed myocardial infarction. Clinical and necropsy observations including quantification of degrees of coronary arterial narrowing. Am J Cardiol 1980;46:754–763.
8. Virmani R, Roberts WC. Non-fatal healed transmural myocardial infarction and fatal non-cardiac disease. Qualification and quantification of coronary arterial narrowing and of left ventricular scarring in 18 necropsy patients. Br Heart J 1981;45:434–441.
9. Tadavarthy SM, Voldaver Z, Edwards JE. Coronary atherosclerosis in subjects with mitral stenosis. Circulation 1976;54:519–521.
10. Befeler B, Kamen AR, Macleod CA. Coronary artery disease and left ventricular function in mitral stenosis. Chest 1970;57:435–439.
11. Lacy J, Goodin R, McMartin D, Masden R, Flowers N. Coronary atherosclerosis in valvular heart disease. Ann Thorac Surg 1977;23:429–435.
12. Chun PKC, Gertz E, Davia JE, Cheitlin MD. Coronary atherosclerosis in mitral stenosis. Chest 1982;81:36–41.
13. Saltups A. Coronary arteriography in isolated aortic and mitral valve disease. Aust NZ J Med 1982;12:494–497.
14. Ramsdale DR, Bennett DH, Bray CL, Ward C, Beton DC, Faragher EB. Angina, coronary risk factors and coronary artery disease in patients with valvular disease. A prospective study. European Heart J 1984;5:716–726.
15. Czer LSC, Gray RJ, Derobertis MA, Bateman TM, Stewart ME, Chaux A, Matloff JM. Mitral valve replacement: impact of coronary artery disease and determinants of prognosis after revascularization. Circulation 1984;70:suppl I:I-198–I-207.
16. Mattina CJ, Green SJ, Tortolani AJ, Padmanabhan VT, Ong LY, Hall MH, Pizzarello RA. Frequency of angiographically significant coronary artery disease in mitral stenosis. Am J Cardiol 1986;57:802–805.

Huge, Unattached Left Atrial Thrombus in Mitral Stenosis

C. S. ROBERTS, M.D., W. C. ROBERTS, M.D.

Surgery and Pathology Branches, National Heart, Lung, and Blood Institute, National Institutes of Health, Bethesda, Maryland, USA

Summary: We describe certain clinical and morphologic findings in a 75-year-old woman in whom a large, spherical, nonadherent, clinically undetected thrombus developed in the left atrium in association with mitral stenosis.

Key words: left atrial thrombus, mitral stenosis, atrial fibrillation, abdominal aortic aneurysm

Introduction

While thrombus isolated to the appendage of the left atrium is common, its presence in the body of the left atrium is infrequent, occurring nearly always in association with mitral stenosis. When thrombus is located in the body of the left atrium and attached to its mural endocardium, similar attached thrombus is virtually always present in the appendage. Nonadherent thrombus in the body of the left atrium is rare, and when it occurs, thrombus is usually absent in the appendage. Wood,[1] in 1814, observed at necropsy an unattached, spherical thrombus in the left atrial body of a 15-year-old girl with mitral stenosis. Abramson,[2] in 1924, found 19 reported necropsy cases aged 15 to 49 years (mean 36) of unattached left atrial thrombus and all 19 patients had associated mitral stenosis. In the

last 35 years, only 3 cases of unattached left atrial body thrombus observed at necropsy have been reported. In 1955, Read and associates[3] described a 62-year-old man with a spherical 5 cm left atrial thrombus without associated mitral stenosis. In 1976, Lie and Entman[4] described an 83-year-old woman with a 3.8 cm spherical left atrial thrombus with associated mitral stenosis. In 1981, Söogaard[5] reported a 76-year-old woman with a 4.5 cm left atrial thrombus without associated mitral stenosis. The rarity of unattached left atrial body thrombus prompted the present report.

Case Report

LC, a 75-year-old white woman, who had acute rheumatic fever at age 20 years, was well until age 60 when atrial fibrillation and systemic hypertension were detected. Soon thereafter she had a stroke, resulting in permanent right hemiplegia. At age 75 she had acute onset of aphasia. On examination the next day, she was obese and semiconscious (responded only to painful stimuli). Blood pressure was 140/90 mmHg and arterial pulse was 100 beats/min. A grade 1/6 systolic precordial murmur was recorded. No diastolic precordial murmur was described. The patient's legs were cool and pale and no femoral, popliteal, dorsalis pedal, or posterior tibial arterial pulses were palpated. The electrocardiogram showed atrial flutter with 2:1 atrioventricular block, left anterior hemiblock, and nonspecific ST-segment changes. Translumbar aortogram showed near complete occlusion of the aorta at the level of the renal arteries and distally. She was anuric and acidotic. Bilateral femoral endarterectomy was performed and peritoneal dialysis started, but she died 6 days later.

At necropsy, the heart weighted 500 g. Both atria were dilated. The myocardium was free of grossly visible foci of necrosis or fibrosis. The tricuspid, pulmonic, and aortic valves were normal. The mitral leaflets and chordae

Address for reprints:

Charles Stewart Roberts, M.D.
Surgery Branch
National Heart, Lung and Blood Institute
National Institutes of Health
Bethesda, MD 20892, USA

Received: November 7, 1989
Accepted with revision: January 2, 1990

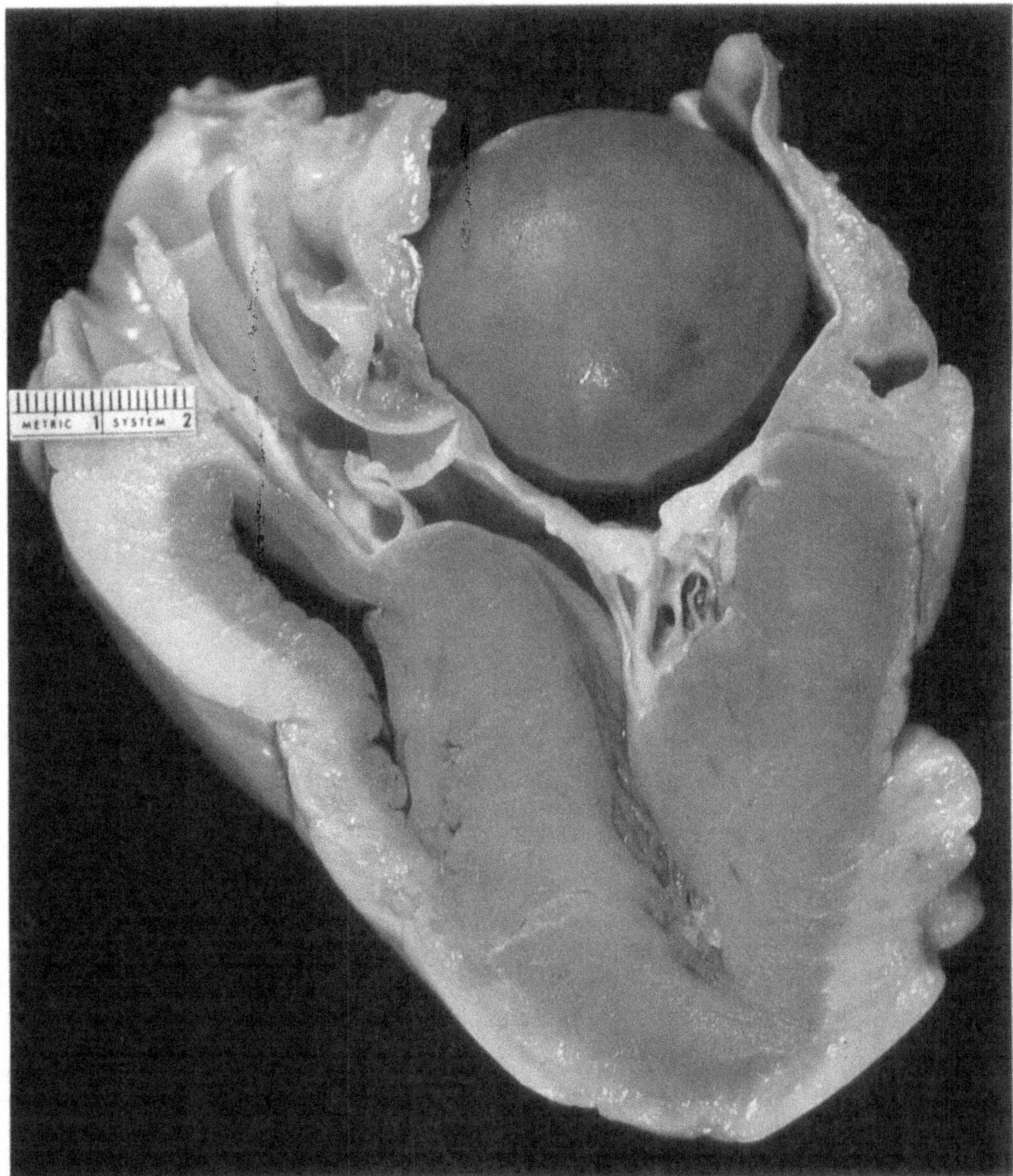

FIG. 1. Longitudinal view of heart showing the large unattached, smooth-surfaced thrombus in the left atrial chamber and a stenotic mitral valve. The left ventricular cavity is not dilated but its wall is thicker than normal.

tendineae were diffusely fibrotic and the mitral orifice was severely stenotic (Figs. 1, 2). The body of the left atrium contained a nonadherent, smooth-surfaced, spherical thrombus weighing 53 g and measuring 4.6 cm in diameter. The abdominal aorta was severely atherosclerotic and aneurysmal, and its lumen was filled with thrombus which obstructed the ostia of both renal arteries, the inferior mesenteric artery, and both common iliac arteries (Fig. 3). Both kidneys had multiple cortical infarcts.

An old infarct was found in the left cerebral hemisphere. (It is likely that the thrombi in these various systemic arteries were not embolic in nature.)

Discussion

The most unusual features of the aforementioned patient are the huge size of the left atrial thrombus and its

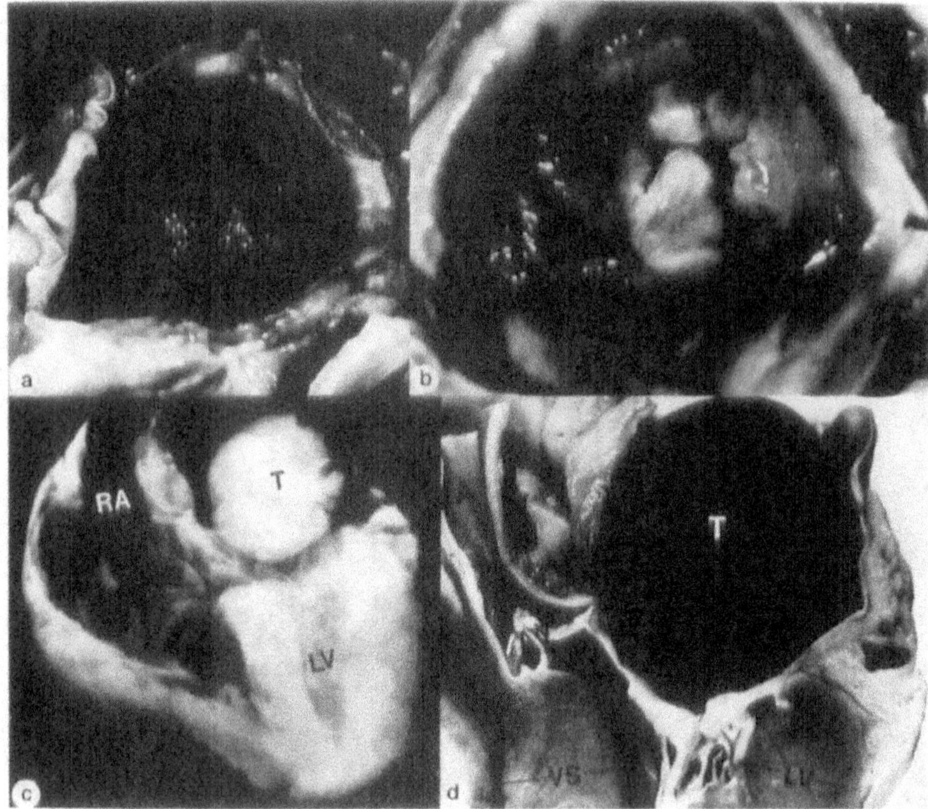

FIG. 2. (A) View of thrombus from above after incising the wall from a right pulmonary vein to a left pulmonary vein. (B) View of opened left atrium from above after removing the thrombus. The valve is stenotic and the mural endocardium is smooth. (C) Radiograph of the heart at necropsy showing the four chambers and the left atrial thrombus. RA = right atrial cavity; RV = right ventricular cavity; T = thrombus. (D) Longitudinal view of left side of the heart after cutting the thrombus in half. The thrombus histologically consisted virtually entirely of fibrin. Ao = aorta; LV = left ventricular wall; VS = ventricular septum.

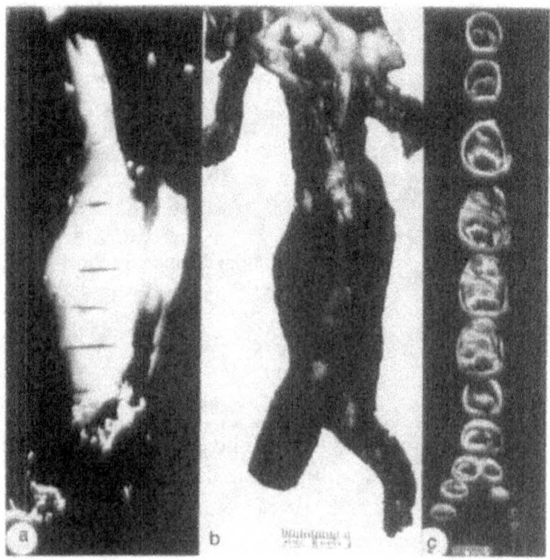

FIG. 3. Abdominal aorta. (A) Radiograph of the abdominal aorta showing an aneurysm, intraaneurysmal thrombus-narrowed lumen, and calcific deposits. (B) Abdominal aorta itself. (C) Transverse sections of the abdominal aorta showing the narrowed lumen due entirely to thrombus.

nonadherence to left atrial endocardium. There were no left atrial endocardial lesions to suggest that the thrombus had at one time been attached. We have never observed thrombus in the body of left atrium, in contrast to that in appendage only, without associated mitral stenosis, but most thrombi in this chamber, of course, are attached to its mural endocardium. How the left atrial thrombus in the present patient could have developed to such a large size without its ever having become attached is unknown.

References

1. Wood W: Letter enclosing the history and dissection of a case in which a foreign body was found within the heart. *Edinburgh Med Surg J* 10, 50 (1814)

2. Abramson JL: Ball thrombi of the heart. *Ann Clin Med* 3, 327 (1924)

3. Read JL, Porter RR, Russi S, Kriz JR: Occlusive avricular thrombi. *Circulation* 12, 250 (1955)

4. Lie JT, Entman ML: ''Hole-in-one'' sudden death: Mitral stenosis and left atrial ball thrombus. *Am Heart J* 91, 798 (1976)

5. Söogaard PE: Free ball thrombus of the left atrium. *Eur J Cardiol* 12, 177 (1981)

Primary Sarcoma of the Heart Causing Mitral Stenosis

Michael J. Domanski, MD, Thomas F. Delaney, MD, David E. Kleiner, Jr., MD, Mary Goswitz, MD, Arthur Agatston, MD, Eben Tucker, MD, Michael Johnson, MD, and William C. Roberts, MD

Cardiac sarcomas are rare and mitral stenosis caused by this neoplasm in the left atrium is even rarer. Such was the case, however, in the patient to be described herein.

A 46-year-old woman (CC no. 22-72-58-1) who died on January 7, 1990, had been well until April 1989, when she had an episode of dizziness and right eye blindness that resolved spontaneously. In June 1989, she had a transient episode of right lower arm numbness and right eye blindness that resolved spontaneous-

From the Cardiology and Pathology Branches, National Heart, Lung, and Blood Institute, the Radiation-Oncology Branch and Laboratory of Pathology, National Cancer Institute, Bethesda, Maryland; the Division of Cardiology, Georgetown University Hospital, Washington, D.C.; the Division of Cardiology, Mount Sinai Medical Center, Miami, Florida; and the National Institutes of Health, Building 10, Room 7B15, Bethesda, Maryland 20892. Manuscript received and accepted May 24, 1990.

ly. In September 1989, she developed orthopnea, dyspnea with walking, syncope and easy fatigability. In October 1989, examination by a cardiologist disclosed a loud first heart sound, a grade 1/6 systolic ejection murmur at the left sternal border and apex that radiated into the axilla and a grade 2/6 systolic murmur at the right sternal border that increased with inspiration. Chest radiograph suggested a dilated left atrium and was consistent with congestive heart failure. An echocardiogram disclosed severe mitral stenosis, mild mitral regurgitation, a dilated right atrium and right ventricle, pericardial effusion and a large mass in the region of the posterior mitral leaflet protruding into and obstructing the mitral orifice (Figure 1). Cardiac catheterization revealed the following pressures (in mm Hg): right atrial mean, 20; right ventricular, 105/18; pulmonary ar-

tery wedge mean, 35; left ventricular, 125/18; and aortic, 125/80. The pulmonary artery wedge—left ventricular mean diastolic gradient was 20 mm Hg. The left ventricle contracted normally. By angiography, neither mitral nor aortic valve regurgitation was present and the epicardial coronary arteries were normal. Thoracotomy was performed and a "lemon"-sized mass involving the basal portion of the left ventricular wall was found. Computed tomography after operation localized the mass to the region of the posterior mitral leaflet. Electrocardiogram showed changes of right ventricular hypertrophy, incomplete right bundle branch block and left atrial abnormality. Echocardiogram showed a large mass in the region of the mitral valve and it extended into the left atrium and left ventricle. By Doppler, the estimated mean mitral pressure gradient was 18 mm Hg. Magnetic resonance imaging (Figure 2) confirmed these findings. The patient received radiation therapy, but died suddenly.

At necropsy (A90-2), the heart with the neoplasm weighed 530 g. The visceral and parietal pericardia

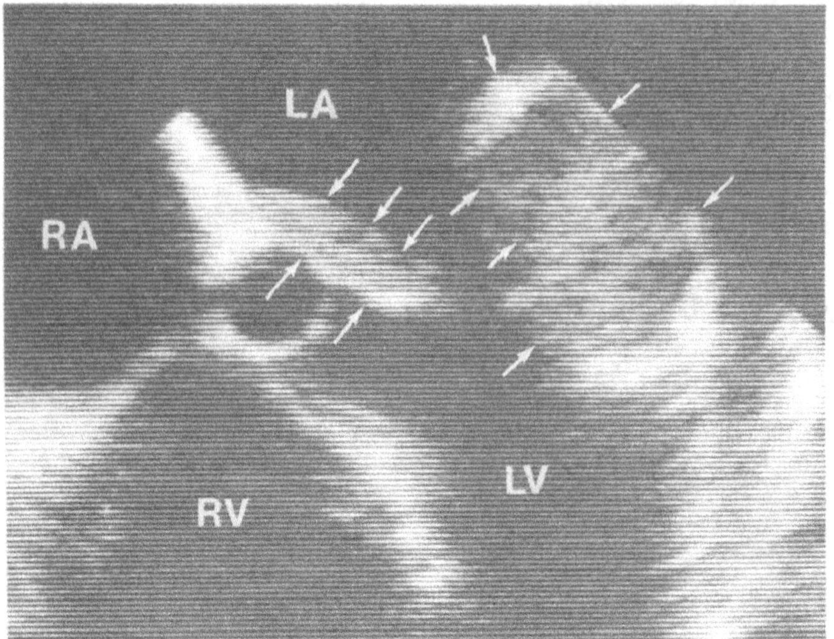

FIGURE 1. Transesophageal echocardiogram showing the tumors *(arrows)* in the left atrial (LA) wall. LV = left ventricle; RA = right atrium; RV = right ventricle.

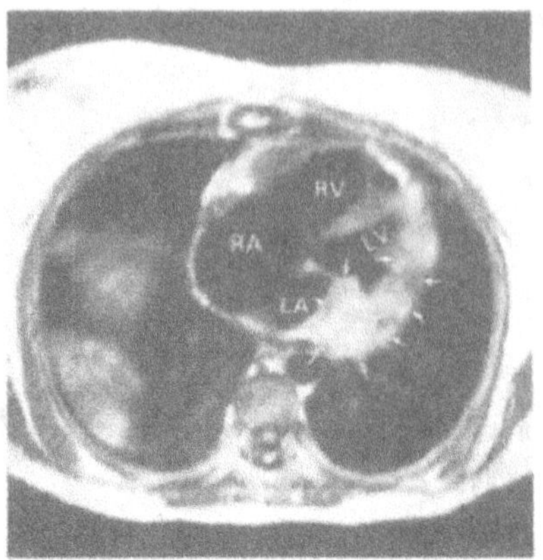

FIGURE 2. Magnetic resonance image of thorax showing the tumor in the walls of left atrium (LA) and left ventricle (LV) and pulmonary infarcts in 1 lung from occlusion of several pulmonary arteries by sarcoma from the right atrium. Abbreviations as in Figure 1.

were adhered to one another by fibrous and neoplastic adhesions. The neoplasm in the wall of the left atrium caused severe obstruction to the mitral orifice (Figure 3) and also to the left pulmonary veins. The neoplasm also invaded the coronary sinus, basal portion of the left ventricular wall and a single tumor deposit was present in the right atrial cavity at the orifice of the coronary sinus. The only body organ containing the neoplasm other than the heart was the lung; a tumor was present in several pulmonary arteries with resulting pulmonary infarcts. Histologically, the neoplasm was a spindle-cell sarcoma. Both pleural spaces (approximately 1,000 ml each) and the peritoneal cavity (1,400 ml) contained dark, amber-colored watery fluid.

The aforementioned patient had sarcoma involving the left atrium and the tumor extended into the mitral orifice producing severe mitral stenosis. We found 7 previously reported cases of left atrial sarcoma causing mitral stenosis and pertinent observations in them are listed in Table I.[1–7] Only 1 of the previously reported cases had the mitral obstruction confirmed by catheterization,

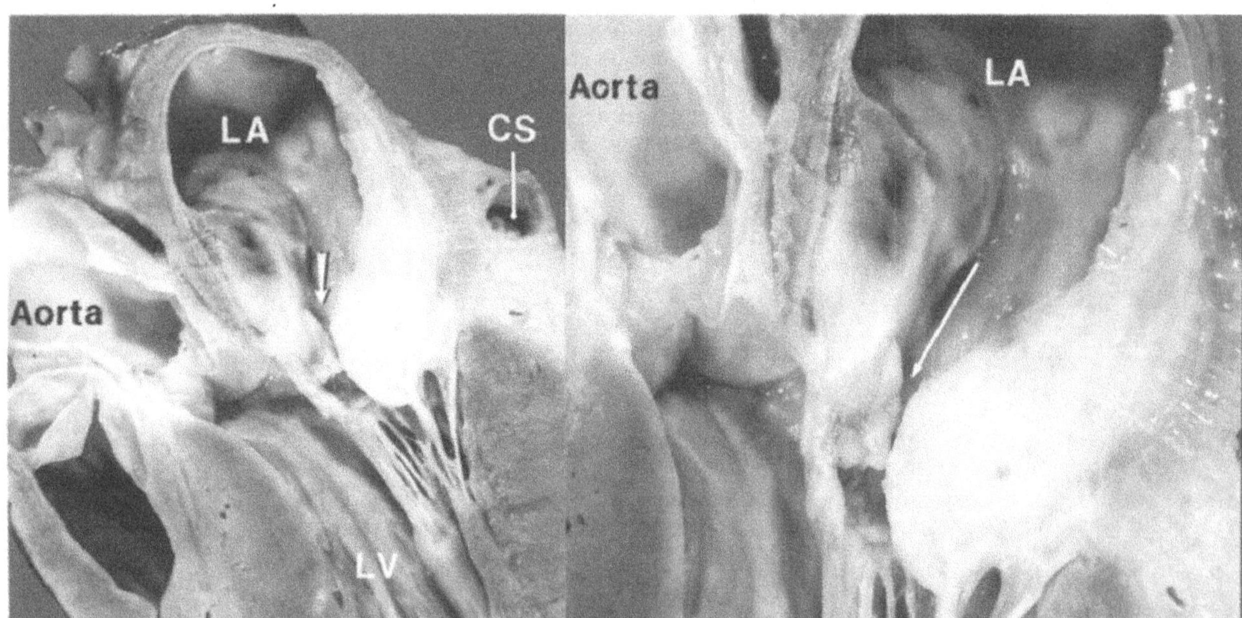

FIGURE 3. Photographs of longitudinal views of the heart showing large tumor deposits in the wall of left atrium (LA) with resulting severe obstruction *(arrows)* to the mitral valve orifice. Tumor also invaded the coronary sinus (CS). Abbreviations as in Figure 1.

TABLE I Observations in Previously Reported Patients with Left Atrial Sarcoma Causing Mitral Stenosis

Case	First Author	Year	Age (yr) & Sex	Duration of Symptoms (months)	DM	OS	P_2	PAW-LV MDG (mm Hg)	Echocardiographic Evidence of MS	Type of Sarcoma
1	Muir	1966	50 F	3	0	—	—	—	—	Chondrosarcoma
2	Dutschmann	1974	39 F	7	+ (4/6)	+	+	—	—	Rhabdomyosarcoma
3	Shuh	1978	37* F		+ (2/6)	+	+	—	—	Fibrous histiocytoma
4	Frendsen	1981	39 F	0.5	+	—	—	—	—	Mesenchymoma
5	Terashima	1983	27 F	5	—	—	—	—	—	Fibrous histiocytoma
6	Ormerod	1984	48 M	"Weeks"	+	—	—	—	+	Angiosarcoma
7	Villasenor	1985	82 F		+ (2/6)	+	—	28	+	Rhabdomyosarcoma

* Only patient still alive at follow-up.
DM = diastolic murmur; LV = left ventricle; MDG = mean diastolic gradient; MS = mitral stenosis; OS = opening snap; PAW = pulmonary arterial wedge; P_2 = pulmonary component of second heart sound; ↑ = increased; + = present; 0 = negative; — = no informatiion.

but all had clear anatomic evidence of mitral obstruction by the neoplasm. Another unusual feature of this sarcoma was invasion of the coronary sinus by the neoplasm and migration (embolization) of the neoplasm from the lumen of the coronary sinus into the right atrium. Portions of the right atrial tumor migrated into several peripheral pulmonary arteries (another embolism), causing neoplastic pulmonary infarcts.

1. Muir CS, Seah CS. Primary chondrosarcomatous mesenchymoma of the mitral valve. *Thorax 1966; 21:254–262.*
2. Dutschmann L, Duarte S, Da Costa JN. Rhabdomyosarcoma of the heart (a case of unusual localization). *Angiology 1974;25:186–196.*
3. Shah AA, Churg A, Sbarbarao JA, Shepard JM, Lamberti J. Malignant fibrous histiocytoma of the heart presenting atrial myxoma. *Cancer 1978;42: 2466–2471.*
4. Frandsen NE, Andersen G, Nielsen JR. Malignant mesenchymoma of the heart presenting as mitral stenosis. *Acta Med Scand 1981;209:235–237.*
5. Terashima T, Aoyama K, Nihei K, Nito T, Imai Y, Takahashi K, Shichibei D. Malignant fibrous histiocytoma of the heart. *Cancer 1983;52:1919– 1926.*
6. Omerod OJ, Spratt PM, Lewis NP, Wallwork J. Primary angiosarcoma of the heart mimicking a left atrial myxoma. *Thorax 1984;39:798–799.*
7. Villasenor HR, Fuentes F, Walker WE. Left atrial rhabdomyosarcoma mimicking mitral valve stenosis. *Tex Heart Inst J 1985;12:107–110.*

Mitral "Annular" Calcium Forming a Complete Circle "O" Causing Mitral Stenosis in Association With a Stenotic Congenitally Bicuspid Aortic Valve and Severe Coronary Artery Disease

Kevin P. Theleman, MD;[1,3] Paul A. Grayburn, MD;[1,3] William C. Roberts, MD[1,2,3]

From the Departments of Medicine (Division of Cardiology)[1] and Pathology[2] and the Baylor Heart and Vascular Institute,[3] Baylor University Medical Center, Dallas, TX

Address for correspondence: William C. Roberts, MD, Baylor Heart and Vascular Institute, Baylor University Medical Center, 621 North Hall Street, Suite H-030, Dallas, TX 75226

E-mail: wcroberts@baylorhealth.edu

Calcific deposits in the epicardial arteries, mitral valve annulus, and aortic valve cusps are common in older persons in the Western world.[1] Recently, we encountered a patient with massive mitral annular calcium causing mitral stenosis in association with a stenotic congenitally bicuspid aortic valve and heavy coronary calcific deposits. The extent of the cardiac calcific deposits is unusual and prompted this report.

A 73-year-old man had an orthotopic liver transplant for alcoholic cirrhosis at age 60, a renal transplant at age 65, a dual-chamber pacemaker inserted for sick sinus syndrome at age 72, and had corticosteroid-induced diabetes mellitus and systemic hypertension. The present examination was prompted by the recent onset of pedal edema. A grade 2/6 systolic ejection murmur that was loudest over the right base of the precordium was present. His body mass index was 22 kg/m². Echocardiography disclosed a 6-mm Hg mean diastolic gradient at the mitral orifice and a left ventricular ejection fraction of about 55% (Figure 1). Cardiac catheterization revealed a peak systolic pressure gradient between the left ventricle and aorta of 50 mm Hg (mean gradient, 38 mm Hg) and an aortic valve area of 0.6 cm². The left anterior descending artery was narrowed up to 70% in

diameter proximally, the second diagonal artery up to 80% proximally, and the ramus intermedius artery up to 80% proximally. The left main coronary artery was widely patent. The dominant left circumflex artery was narrowed up to 50% in diameter and was heavily calcified. The nondominant right coronary artery was free of narrowing.

The aortic valve was replaced with a 21-mm Medtronic Mosaic (Medtronic, Inc., Mineapolis, MN) bioprosthesis. The surgically removed aortic valve was congenitally bicuspid (Figure 2). Aortosaphenous vein grafts were placed to the left anterior descending and the first marginal coronary arteries. An intra-aortic balloon pump was placed intraoperatively. Aortic cross-clamp time was 149 minutes. The postoperative course was complicated by the low cardiac output syndrome, and death occurred 5 days postoperatively.

At necropsy, the coronary arteries and mitral annular region were massively calcified (Figure 3). The ventricular cavities were not dilated (Figure 4). The bioprosthesis in the aortic valve position appeared to have functioned normally. The venous conduits to the left anterior descending and obtuse marginal arteries were patent.

The most prevalent site of cardiac calcific deposits is the epicardial coronary arteries, followed by the mitral annular area and aortic valve cusps. The apical portions of the left papillary

 **www.lejacq.com**   **ID: 5261**

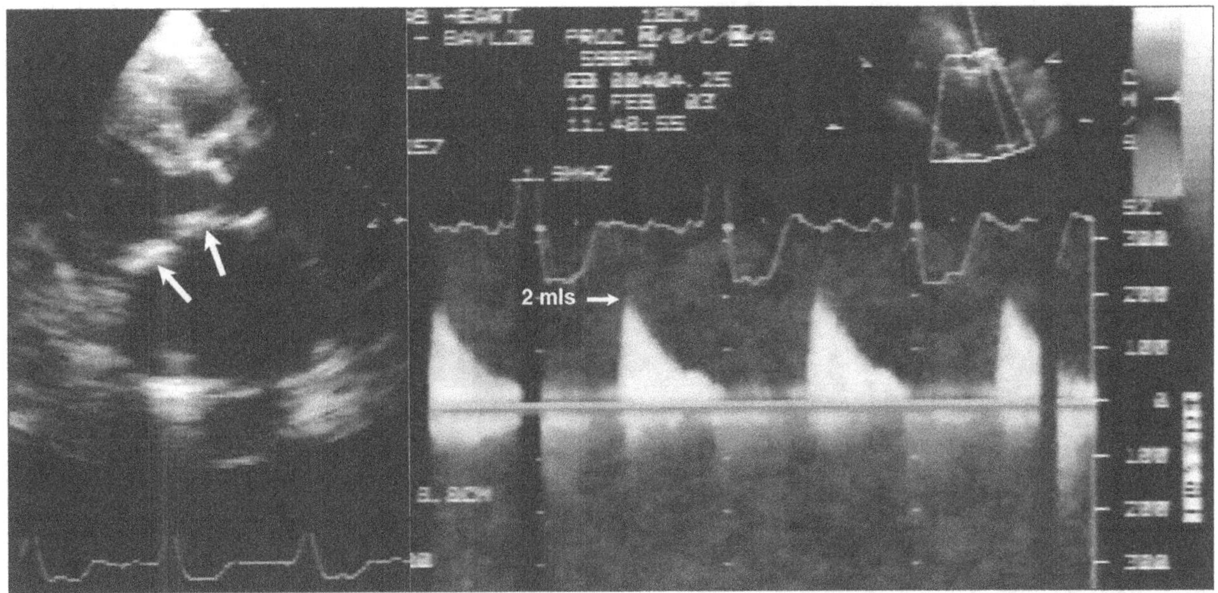

Figure 1. Echocardiogram. Left panel: parasternal long-axis view showing extensive calcification deposits of the mitral annulus (arrows) and aortic valve; right panel: transmitral Doppler inflow showing a peak velocity of 2.0 m/sec and a mean gradient of 6 mm Hg

muscles are the fourth most common area of the heart to have calcific deposits.[1] The term "mitral annular calcium" is not accurate in that the calcium deposits are actually located between the ventricular surface of the posterior mitral valve leaflet and the mural endocardium of the left ventricle. When the calcium deposits are extensive, a "C"-shaped or "J"-shaped configuration can appear on radiograph. In rare cases, the calcium extends across the anterior mitral leaflet forming an "O"-shaped configuration.[2] Mitral annular calcium is often associated with mild or moderate mitral regurgitation, but severe regurgitation due to the calcium deposits alone probably does not occur.[2] Significant mitral stenosis due to annular calcium has been reported only in the setting of left ventricular outflow obstruction, as occurred in the present patient.[3]

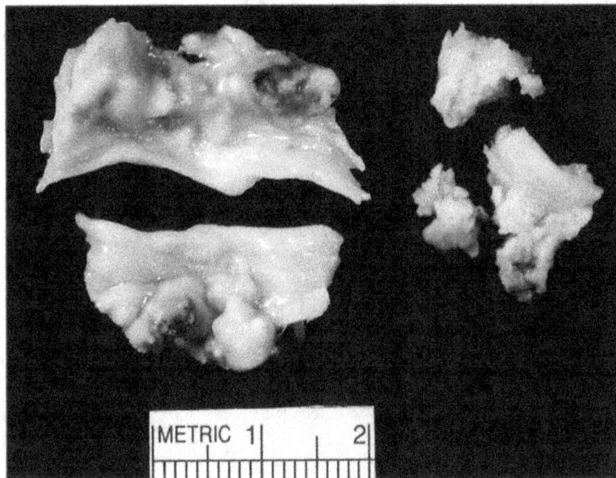

Figure 2. Photograph of the operatively excised focally calcified, stenotic, congenitally bicuspid aortic valve

forming a complete circle or "O" configuration: clinical and necropsy observations. *Am Heart J.* 1981;101:619–621.

REFERENCES

1 Roberts WC. The senile cardiac calcification syndrome. *Am J Cardiol.* 1986;58:572–574.
2 Roberts WC, Waller BF. Mitral valve "annular" calcium
3 Hammer WJ, Roberts WC, deLeon AC. "Mitral stenosis" secondary to combined "massive" mitral annular calcific deposits and small, hypertrophied left ventricles. Hemodynamic documentation in four patients. *Am J Med.* 1978;64:371–376.

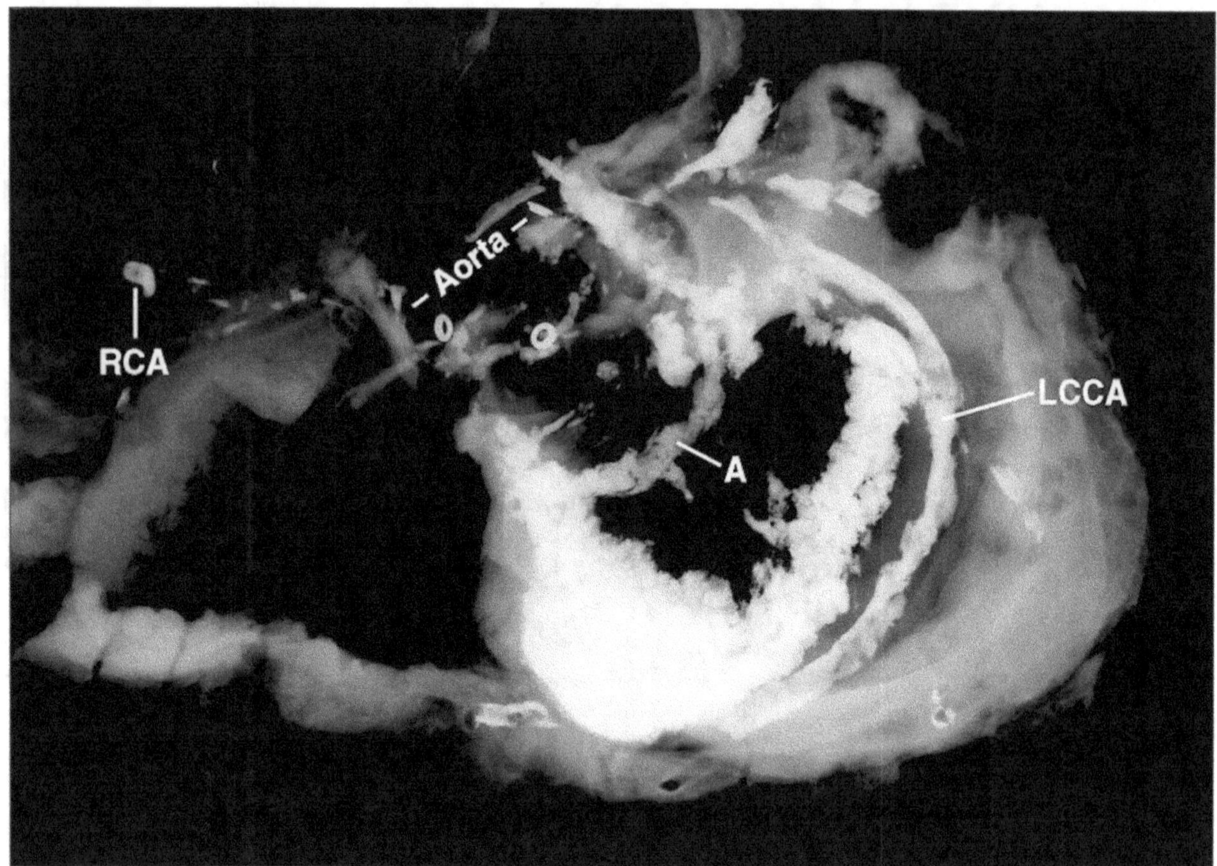

Figure 3. Radiograph of the heart at necropsy. A huge amount of calcium is located beneath the posterior mitral leaflet and extends across the anterior (A) mitral leaflet forming a circle "O." The left circumflex coronary artery (LCCA) is heavily and diffusely calcified (about 50% of patients with a congenitally bicuspid aortic valve have a dominant left circumflex rather than a dominant right coronary artery [RCA], the situation in about 90% of patients with a tricuspid aortic valve). Calcific deposits also are present in the left main and left anterior descending coronary arteries.

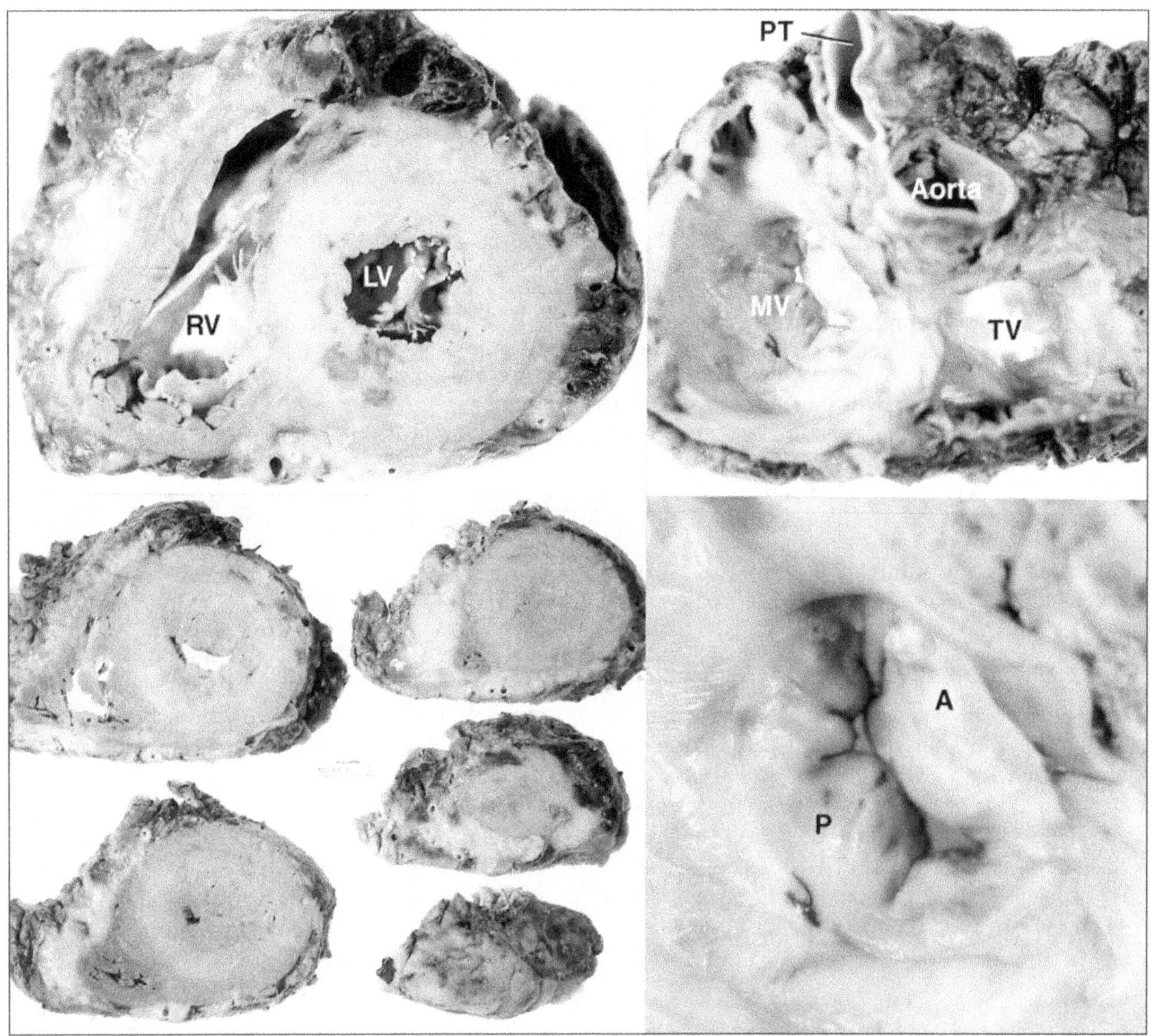

Figure 4. Photographs of the heart at necropsy. Upper left: view of left (LV) and right (RV) ventricles showing normal-sized cavities and a small area of myocardial necrosis in the posterior wall; lower left: transverse sections of the cardiac ventricles showing small cavities and no myocardial lesions; upper right: view of mitral (MV) and tricuspid valve (TV) orifices from the atrial aspects, with pulmonary trunk (PT); lower right: close-up view of the MV from the left atrium showing the anterior (A) and posterior (P) leaflets

Comparison of Findings in Patients With Versus Without Atrial Fibrillation Just Before Isolated Mitral Valve Replacement for Rheumatic Mitral Stenosis (With or Without Associated Mitral Regurgitation)

John Bryan Sims, MD[a,b], and William Clifford Roberts, MD[a,b,*]

Among 104 patients with mitral stenosis (MS) severe enough or symptomatic enough to warrant mitral valve replacement (MVR), 47 (45%) had atrial fibrillation (AF) and 57 (55%) had sinus rhythm just before the MVR. Of the latter 57 patients, 21 (37%) had had previous episodes compatible with AF. If these 21 patients were included with the 47 patients with electrocardiographic documentation of AF just before MVR, a total of 68 (65%) would have had ≥1 presumed episodes of AF before MVR. The 13 patients with previous mitral commissurotomy had a frequency of AF similar to that of the 91 whose first operation was MVR. Compared with the patients with sinus rhythm just before MVR, those with AF had more heart failure (functional class III or IV preoperatively, 79% vs 62%), larger left atria (6.0 vs 5.2 cm), larger left ventricles in peak systole (4.0 vs 2.6 cm), and more had 2 or 3 coronary arteries narrowed >50% in diameter (23% vs 10%).   © 2006 Elsevier Inc. All rights reserved. (Am J Cardiol 2006;97:1035–1038)

The frequency of atrial fibrillation (AF) is higher in patients with mitral stenosis (MS) than in any other condition. In a study of 710 patients with unoperated MS seen in an outpatient clinic by Diker and associates[1] and unassociated with aortic valve disease, 343 (48%) had AF by electrocardiogram. The average age of those with chronic AF was 43 years and those with sinus rhythm, 33 years. The present study focuses on patients with MS who underwent mitral valve replacement (MVR) and compares those with AF to those without AF by electrocardiogram immediately before MVR.

• • •

Patients having isolated (no other cardiac valves replaced) MVR for MS at Baylor University Medical Center from May 1993 to January 2005 were reviewed. All operatively excised stenotic mitral valves submitted to the surgical pathology department during this period were examined by 1 of us (WCR). That the valves were stenotic was determined by gross examination of the operatively excised valve by 1 of us (WCR), and by examining the clinical and hemodynamic records to confirm the presence of MS with or without mitral regurgitation . Patients ≤20 years of age and patients having simultaneous aortic and/or tricuspid valve replacement were excluded. Cases in whom the MS was the result of mitral annular calcium also were excluded.

A total of 104 patients had MVR for MS (with or without mitral regurgitation) during the 128-month period of this study. Electrocardiographic data immediately before MVR were available in all patients. Echocardiographic data were available in 65 patients (63%), hemodynamic data in 74 patients (71%), and coronary arterial angiographic data in 91 patients (88%).

Statistical analysis was performed using SigmaStat (version 2.0; SPSS, Inc., Chicago, Illinois). Parametric tests were used for the analysis of the data, which passed the assumption tests for normality and equal variance: for continuous variables, unpaired t test was performed for 2 variable comparisons and 1-way analysis of variance for >2 variable comparisons. When the data did not pass the assumption tests, nonparametric tests, i.e., Man-Whitney Rank Sum test for 2 variable comparisons and Kruskal-Wallis 1-way analysis of variance on ranks test for >2 continuous variable comparisons, were used. To compare the percentages in 2 different groups, the z-test was used. To compare the percentages in >3 different groups, the chi-square test was used. A p value <0.05 was considered statistically significant.

Table 1 compares certain clinical, echocardiograpic, hemodynamic, and cineangiographic findings in the 13 patients with previous mitral commissurotomy to the 91 patients without previous mitral commissurotomy. The only difference observed between these 2 groups were higher pressures in the aorta in those with previous mitral commissurotomy versus those whose first mitral operation was MVR.

Table 2 excludes the 13 patients with previous mitral commissurotomy and compares the remaining 91 patients whose first cardiac operation was MVR. The 38 patients (42%) who had AF by electrocardiogram immediately before MVR compared with the 53 patients (58%) who were in sinus rhythm immediately before MVR had a higher

From the Departments of [a]Internal Medicine (Division of Cardiology) and [b]Pathology, and the Baylor Heart & Vascular Institute, Baylor University Medical Center, Dallas, Texas. Manuscript received October 11, 2005; revised manuscript received and accepted November 15, 2005.

* Corresponding author: Tel: 214-820-7911; fax: 212-820-7533.
E-mail address: wc.roberts@baylorhealth.edu (W.C. Roberts).

Table 1

Comparison of various variables in the 13 patients with previous mitral commissurotomy to the 91 patients without mitral commissurotomy

| | Previous Mitral Commissurotomy | | |
Variable	No (n = 91)	Yes (n = 13)	p Value
Age (years)	33–80 (60)	35–70 (54)	0.09
White	63 (69%)	6 (46%)	0.49
Female	79 (87%)	12 (92%)	0.98
Atrial fibrillation immediately before mitral valve replacement by electrocardiogram	38 (42%)	9 (69%)	0.28
Atrial fibrillation (by history)	57 (62%)	10 (77%)	0.58
Systemic hypertension (by history)	48 (53%)	4 (31%)	0.75
Diabetes mellitus	15 (16%)	2 (15%)	0.32
Prior myocardial infarction	8 (8%)		0.42
Coronary bypass at time of mitral operation	23 (25%)	1 (8%)	0.23
New York Heart Association functional class			
I	1 (1%)		
II	27 (30%)	1 (8%)	
III	58 (64%)	12 (92%)	
IV	5 (5%)		
Number of major coronary arteries narrowed >50% in diameter			0.80
0	64 (70%)	10 (77%)	
1	14 (5%)	2 (15%)	
2	5 (5%)	1 (8%)	
3	6 (7%)	0 (0%)	
Left main	2 (2%)	0 (0%)	
Body mass index (kg/m^2): range (mean)	16–84 (30)	17–34 (26)	0.51
<25	34 (37%)	5 (85%)	0.21
26–30	31 (34%)	7 (54%)	
<30	26 (29%)	1 (8%)	
Days in hospital after mitral operation	4–36 (9)	5–18 (8)	0.25
Echocardiographic data: range (mean)			
Left atrium (mm)	38–66 (52)	45–92 (60)	0.08
Left ventricle, peak systole (mm)	20–52 (34)	32–42 (37)	0.73
Mitral valve area (cm^2)	0.7–1.6 (1.2)	0.8–1.6 (1.1)	0.14
Ejection fraction (%)	10–70 (56)	50–65 (59)	0.59
Cardiovascular direct pressures (mm Hg): range (mean)			
Mean diastolic gradient between pulmonary artery wedge and left ventricle	5–35 (16)	10–26 (15)	0.90
Pulmonary artery wedge	12–60 (25)	15–35 (23)	0.65
Right ventricular peak systole	27–170 (58)	30–64 (45)	0.09
Right ventricular end-diastole	1–36 (13)	12–14 (13)	0.86
Right atrium mean	1–35 (11)	8–12 (10)	0.84
Pulmonary artery peak systole	24–171 (55)	26–68 (46)	0.21
Pulmonary artery end-diastole	7–76 (25)	15–26 (20)	0.18
Pulmonary artery mean	13–115 (37)	21–40 (30)	0.10
Left ventricular systole	85–184 (129)	106–176 (140)	0.31
Left ventricular end-diastole	4–72 (15)	6–50 (21)	0.34
Aorta peak systole	90–179 (127)	125–187 (148)	0.04
Aorta end-diastole	32–100 (71)	70–90 (82)	0.04
Aorta mean	58–142 (96)	96–125 (110)	0.02
Other cardiac catheterization data:			
Valve area (cm^2)	0.5–2.1 (1.0)	0.8–1.2 (1.1)	0.40
Cardiac index (L/min/m^2)	1.5–3.3 (2.3)	1.8–3.2 (2.5)	0.42
Ejection fraction (%)	15–70 (58)	45–60 (54)	0.37
Associated mitral regurgitation	74 (81%)	9 (69%)	0.68
Maze procedure	17 (19%)	1 (8%)	0.29
Tricuspid valve annuloplasty	7 (8%)	2 (15%)	0.29
Patent foramen ovale closure	7 (8%)	2 (15%)	0.29

percentage of heart failure class III or IV (79% vs 62%), a higher percentage of narrowing >50% in diameter of 2 or 3 major epicardial coronary arteries (23% vs 10%), more days in the hospital after MVR (10 vs 9 days), larger left atria (5.7 vs 4.8 cm), larger left ventricular cavities in peak systole (4.0 vs 2.6 cm), smaller mitral valve areas (1.0 vs 1.3 cm), and lower mean pulmonary artery wedge pressures (22 vs 27 mm Hg). Comparison of various variables among the 20 patients who had had a history of an arrhythmia but had sinus rhythm by electrocardiogram immediately before

Table 2

Comparison of clinical findings in patients with and without atrial fibrillation (AF) by electrocardiogram just before mitral valve replacement (MVR) for mitral stenosis and never a previous mitral commissurotomy (n = 104)

Variable	Atrial Fibrillation by Electrocardiogram Immediately Before MVR		
	Yes (n = 38)	No* (n = 53)	p Value
Age (years)	42–80 (62)	33–78 (59)	0.22
White	27 (71%)	36 (68%)	0.098
Female/male	34 (89%)/4 (11%)	45 (85%)/8 (15%)	.098
Systemic hypertension (by history)	20 (53%)	28 (53%)	0.77
Diabetes mellitus	9 (24%)	6 (11%)	0.97
Prior myocardial infarction	5 (13%)	3 (6%)	0.38
Coronary bypass at time of mitral operation	11 (29%)	12 (23%)	0.88
New York Heart Association functional class			
I	0 (0%)	1 (2%)	0.31
II	8 (21%)	19 (36%)	
III	27 (71%)	31 (58%)	0.05
IV	3 (8%)	2 (4%)	
Number of major coronary arteries narrowed >50% in diameter			
0	25 (66%)	35 (66%)	0.14
1	4 (11%)	13 (25%)	
2	5 (12%)	2 (4%)	0.001
3	4 (11%)	3 (6%)	
Left main	1 (3%)	1 (2%)	
Body mass index (kg/m^2): range (mean)	16–43 (28)	16–48 (28)	0.29–0.75
<25	14 (36%)	21 (40%)	
26–30	12 (32%)	19 (36%)	
<30	12 (32%)	13 (25%)	
Days in hospital after mitral operation	4–36 (10)	4–25 (9)	0.03
Echocardiographic data: range (mean)			
Left atrium (mm)	43–60 (57)	33–65 (48)	0.002
Left ventricle, peak systole (mm)	32–52 (40)	20–30 (26)	0.02
Mitral valve area (cm^2)	0.7–1.4 (1.0)	1–1.6 (1.3)	0.007
Ejection fraction (%)	10–70 (54)	30–70 (57)	0.25
Cardiovascular direct pressures (mm Hg): range (mean)			
Mean diastolic gradient between pulmonary artery wedge and left ventricle	5–35 (15)	4–33 (18)	0.13
Pulmonary artery wedge	12–46 (22)	7–60 (27)	0.02
Right ventricular peak systole	27–170 (59)	31–119 (58)	0.61
Right ventricular end-diastole	2–25 (12)	1–46 (14)	0.36
Right atrium mean	3–26 (11)	1–35 (11)	0.77
Pulmonary artery peak systole	24–171 (55)	28–103 (54)	0.68
Pulmonary artery end-diastole	10–76 (27)	7–46 (23)	0.39
Pulmonary artery mean	15–115 (38)	13–64 (37)	0.55
Left ventricular systole	85–163 (125)	82–234 (131)	0.84
Left ventricular end-diastole	4–23 (13)	1–72 (17)	0.14
Aorta peak systole	90–171 (128)	87–225 (126)	0.90
Aorta end-diastole	32–100 (72)	5–100 (71)	0.72
			0.79
Other cardiac catheterization data:			
Mitral valve area (cm^2)	0.5–1.4 (0.9)	0.7–2.1 (1.1)	0.07
Cardiac index (L/min/m^2)	1.5–3.3 (2.2)	1.4–3.4 (2.3)	0.17
Ejection fraction (%)	15–65 (51)	25–70 (58)	0.06
Associated mitral regurgitation	29 (76%)	45 (85%)	0.51
Maze procedure	12 (32%)	5 (9%)	0.70
Tricuspid valve annuloplasty	5 (13%)	4 (8%)	0.40
Patent foramen ovale repair	1 (3%)	4 (8%)	0.04

* Of the 53 patients with sinus rhythm by electrocardiogram immediately before MVR, 20 (38%) had had previous episodes constantly with AF. Comparison of these 20 patients with paroxysmal AF to the 33 without disclosed only 1 significant difference: those with paroxysmal AF had a higher frequency of left atria >4.0 cm than the group who never had AF.

MVR showed only 1 significant difference between them, i.e., a higher percent of left atrial cavities (>4.0 cm) in the paroxysmal AF group by echocardiography.

• • •

The present study showed that among 104 patients with MS, 47 (45%) had AF and 57 (55%) had sinus rhythm by electrocardiogram immediately before MVR. The frequency of electrocardiographically documented AF just before MVR was similar in the 13 patients with previous mitral commissurotomy compared with the 91 patients in whom MVR was their first cardiac operation. Of the 57 patients among the total of 104 with sinus rhythm just before MVR, 21 (37%) had a history of a dysrhythmia, presumably AF. If these 21 patients were included with the 47 with electrocardiographic documentation of AF just before MVR, a total of 68 (65%) would have had ≥1 presumed episodes of AF before MVR.

Others have shown the left atrium to be larger in MS patients with AF compared with those in sinus rhythm. Probst et al[2] studied 135 patients with MS who had not undergone a mitral valve operation: 73 (54%) had AF (intermittent in 27 and persistent in 46) and 62 (46%) had persistent sinus rhythm. Compared with the sinus rhythm group, the AF patients were older (52 vs 42 years), had a higher frequency of "moderate" and "gross" left atrial enlargement by radiograph (41 of 73 [56%] vs 26 of 62 [42%]), and lower cardiac indexes (2.2 vs 2.8 L/min^2). Henry and associates[3] studied, by M-mode echocardiography, 85 patients with "isolated mitral valve disease" (at least 67 of whom had MS) and found AF in 47 (55%), 45 (96%) of whom had left atrial dimensions ≥40 mm. Of 733 unoperated MS patients studied by Diker et al,[1] the left atrial diameter averaged 5.7 ± 1.2 cm among the 355 patients (48%) with AF (unassociated with aortic valve disease) and 4.0 ± 7 cm among the 378 patients (52%) with sinus rhythm. The left atrium usually becomes smaller after a successful operation for MS.[4]

Acknowledgment: We are grateful to Jong Mi Ko, BS, for the superb help with the statistical analyses.

1. Diker E, Aydogdu S, Özdemir M, Kural T, Polat K, Cehreli S, Erdogan A, Göksel S. Prevalence and predictors of atrial fibrillation in rheumatic valvular heart disease. *Am J Cardiol* 1996;77:96–98.
2. Probst P, Goldschlager N, Selzer A. Left atrial size and atrial fibrillation in mitral stenosis. Factors influencing their relationship. *Circulation* 1973;48:1282–1287.
3. Henry WL, Morganroth J, Pearlman AS, Clark CE, Redwood DR, Itscoitz SB, Epstein SE. Relation between echocardiographically determined left atrial size and atrial fibrillation. *Circulation* 1976;53:273–279.
4. Sherrid MV, Clark RD, Cohn K. Echocardiographic analysis of left atrial size before and after operation in mitral valve disease. *Am J Cardiol* 1979;43:171–178.

Mitral Valve Repair for Pure Mitral Regurgitation Followed Years Later by Mitral Valve Replacement for Mitral Stenosis

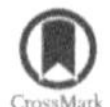

Tiffany M. Becker, BS[a], Paul A. Grayburn, MD[a,b], and William C. Roberts, MD[a,b,c,*]

We describe herein 2 patients who developed severe mitral stenosis (MS) approximately two decades after a mitral valve repair operation for pure mitral regurgitation (MR) secondary to mitral valve prolapse. This report's purpose is to point out that use of a circumferential mitral annular ring during the repair has the potential to produce a transmitral pressure gradient just like that occurring after mitral valve replacement utilizing a mechanical prosthesis or a bioprosthesis in the mitral position. © 2017 Elsevier Inc. All rights reserved. (Am J Cardiol 2017;120:160–166)

Recently, we reported findings in 29 patients who had undergone mitral valve repair operations for pure MR with insertion of an annular ring and later underwent mitral valve replacement for either recurring MR or development of MS or obstruction to left ventricular outflow.[1] The present report was prompted by study of 2 additional patients who developed severe MS many years (≈20) after the repair operation for pure MR due to mitral valve prolapse. Because of the late development of well-documented MS, an infrequently reported occurrence after a repair operation for pure MR, we believe that this additional report is worthwhile.

Patients Described

Pertinent features in each of the 2 patients are summarized in Table 1. At the first operation, patient #1 had a quadrangular resection of a portion of posterior mitral leaflet and ring insertion; patient #2 had the ring insertion but whether a portion of the posterior leaflet was resected is uncertain. The interval between the 2 mitral valve operative procedures was 19 years in patient #1 and 21 years in patient #2. Just before the replacement operation the mean transmitral gradient by echocardiogram was 10 mm Hg in patient #1 and 12 mm Hg in patient #2 (Figures 1 to 3). Computed tomographic imaging in patient #1 showed focal calcific deposits in the mitral leaflets, something not present before the repair operation 19 years earlier (Figure 4). Certain morphologic features of the operatively excised mitral valves and rings are shown in Figures 5 and 6. At early postoperative follow-up both patients were asymptomatic (case #1 four months and case #2 one month postoperatively, respectively).

[a]Baylor Heart and Vascular Institute, [b]Division of Cardiology, Department of Internal Medicine, and [c]Department of Pathology, Baylor University Medical Center, Dallas, Texas. Manuscript received January 3, 2017; revised manuscript received and accepted March 20, 2017.

See page 163 for disclosure information.

*Corresponding author: Tel: (214) 820-7911; fax: (214) 820-7533.

E-mail address: william.roberts1@bswhealth.org (W.C. Roberts).

Table 1

Pertinent clinical and morphologic features in the 2 patients having mitral valve repair for mitral valve prolapse and approximately 20 years later mitral valve replacement for mitral stenosis

Variable	Case	
	#1	#2
1. Age (years) at the mitral repair operation	21	32
2. Age (years) at mitral valve replacement	40	53
3. Interval (years) between the 2 operations	19	21
4. Sex	Man	Woman
5. Atrial Fibrillation	0	+
6. Ventricular arrhythmia	0	+
7. Body mass index (Kg/m^2)	29	35
8. Degree of mitral regurgitation (0-4$^+$)	1$^+$	1$^+$
9. Transvalvular mean gradient (mmHg)*	10	12
10. Mitral area (cm^2) just before mitral replacement*	1.1	1.2
11. Right ventricular peak systolic pressure (mmHg)*	46	— —
12. Left ventricular ejection fraction (%)*	55	45
13. Left atrial cavity size (cm)*	4.7	5.0
14. Left ventricular cavity size*	Normal	Normal
15. Type of mitral ring	Duran (31mm)	Carpentier-Edwards
16. Area (cm^2) enclosed by the operatively excised mitral ring	2.8	3.5
17. Substitute valve inserted (mitral position)	Bioprosthesis (#27)	Mechanical (SJM) (#29)

— — = no information available; SJM = St. Jude Medical.

* By echocardiogram just before the mitral valve replacement operation.

Discussion

Development of MS after a mitral valve repair operation for pure MR using an annular ring may not be a rare occurrence. Indeed, 16 of the 29 patients described in the previously mentioned study developed some degree of MS before the replacement operation.[1] Although nearly

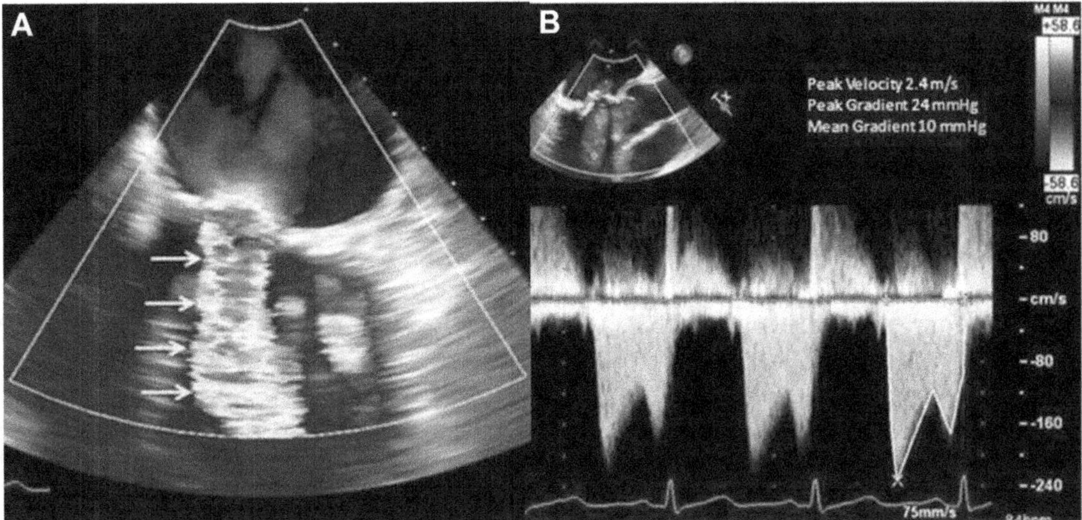

Figure 1. (Case #1) *(A)* Four-chamber view showing markedly turbulent diastolic flow into the left ventricle, characterized by a mosaic color Doppler pattern *(arrows). (B)* Continuous-wave Doppler profile of mitral inflow showing elevated velocities/gradients.

all prosthetic and bioprosthetic substitute valves utilized for mitral valve replacement have an inherent gradient, the 2 patients described herein developed MS many years later, due presumably primarily to late thickening of the valve leaflets and chords. Measurement of the area enclosed by the ring excised at the time of mitral valve replacement, however, indicated that the area was much smaller than that of a normal mitral valve, suggesting at

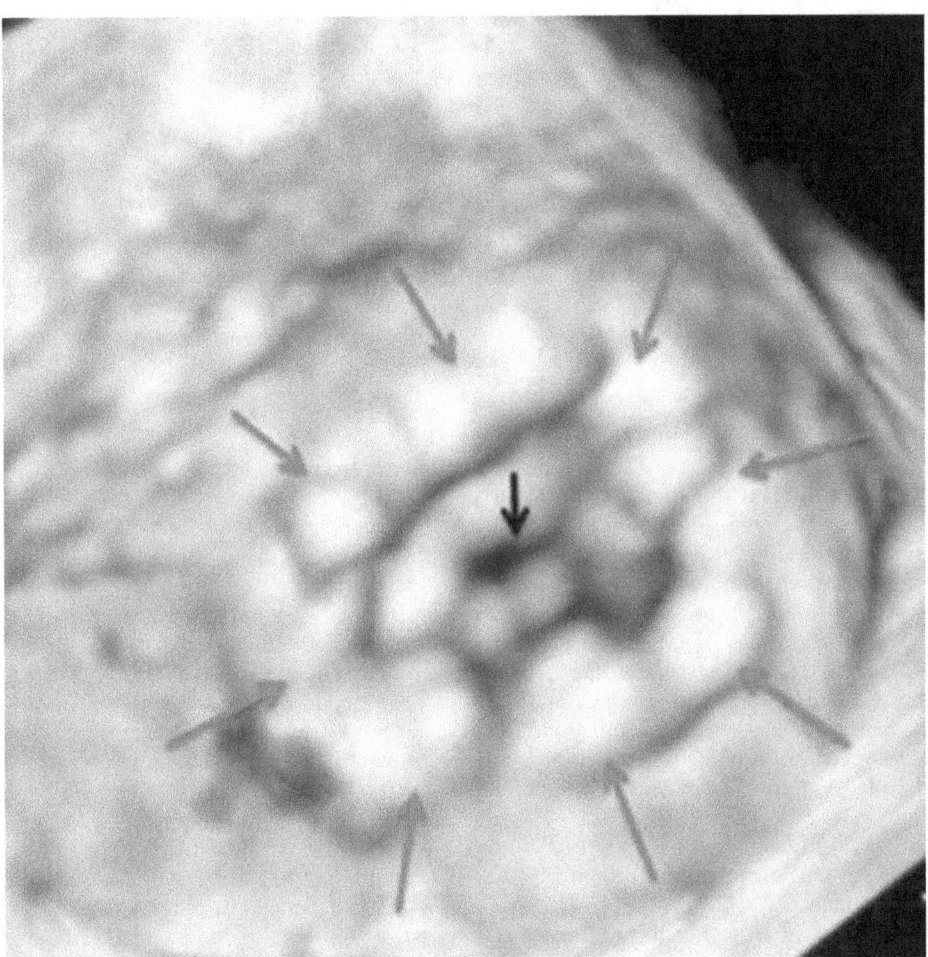

Figure 2. (Case #1) 3D "Surgeon's view" from early diastole showing mitral ring *(blue arrows).* Within the ring, there is thickened leaflet and subvalvular tissue with a small orifice *(black arrow).*

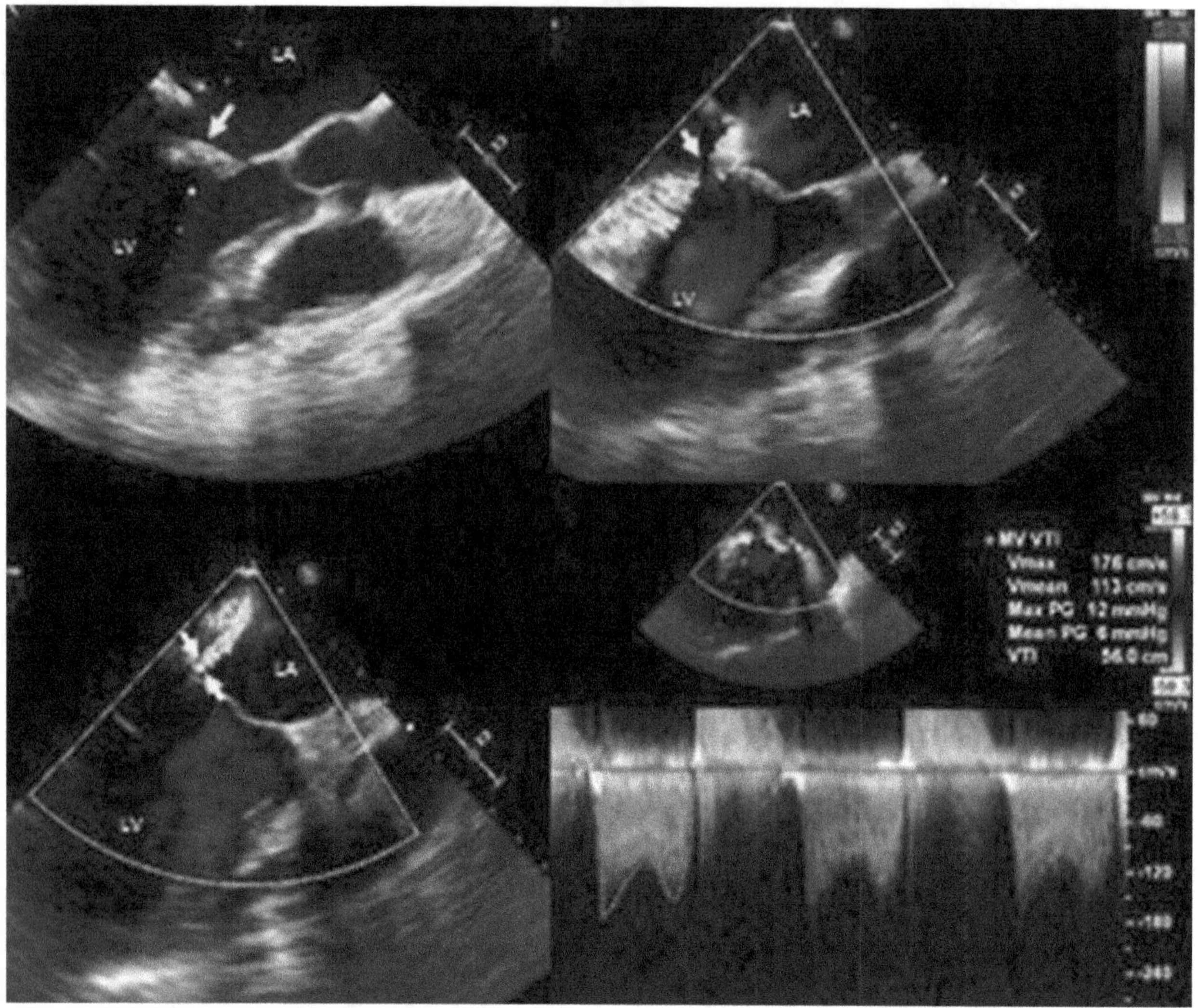

Figure 3. (Case #2) Intraoperative TEE images from the patient. *Top left:* long-axis view showing thickened anterior mitral leaflet *(arrow)*. *Top right:* diastolic frame showing mitral stenosis jet *(arrow)*. *Bottom left:* systolic frame showing mild mitral regurgitation with vena contracta width 3 mm *(arrows)*. *Bottom right:* continuous-wave Doppler velocity profile across the mitral valve showing peak gradient 12 mm Hg and mean gradient 6 mm Hg under anesthesia.

least the possibility that the ring inserted at the time of mitral repair may have been a bit too small for the long term. In both patients after the repair operation the mitral leaflets appeared to "gather" within the ring area, like the gathering at the waist of a woman's skirt, causing focal fibrous thickening of the leaflets due to constant abnormal contact over nearly 20 years. Both patients described were asymptomatic for over 15 years after the repair procedure. Had these 2 patients had the repair operation at age 55 years, the average age of the repair procedure in the previously mentioned report,[1] both may well have died before developing symptoms of mitral dysfunction again.

A number of articles have appeared providing follow-up after a mitral valve repair operation for pure MR, mainly mitral valve prolapse.[2–23] Several of them have mentioned the development of MS after the mitral valve repair operation[3–5,14–17,21–23] (Table 2). The frequency of development of MS according to these published reports is very uncommon. The average age of the mitral repair, however, was in the 50s or 60s such that long follow-up, as in our 2 described patients, may not have been possible. Additionally, echocardiograms are not performed routinely in all these patients, suggesting that the actual frequency of MS perhaps will be much more common than suggested by these reports. In addition to these reports,[3–5,14–17,21–23] which included many patients, at least 5 case studies in adults have appeared in patients developing MS several years after mitral valve repair for pure MR (Table 3).[24–28]

How can the development of MS after mitral repair for pure MR be avoided? One might be to use an annular ring which is not too small. A second might be to use a partial annuloplasty band rather than a circumferential ring. These opinions of course need to be proven to be right or wrong.

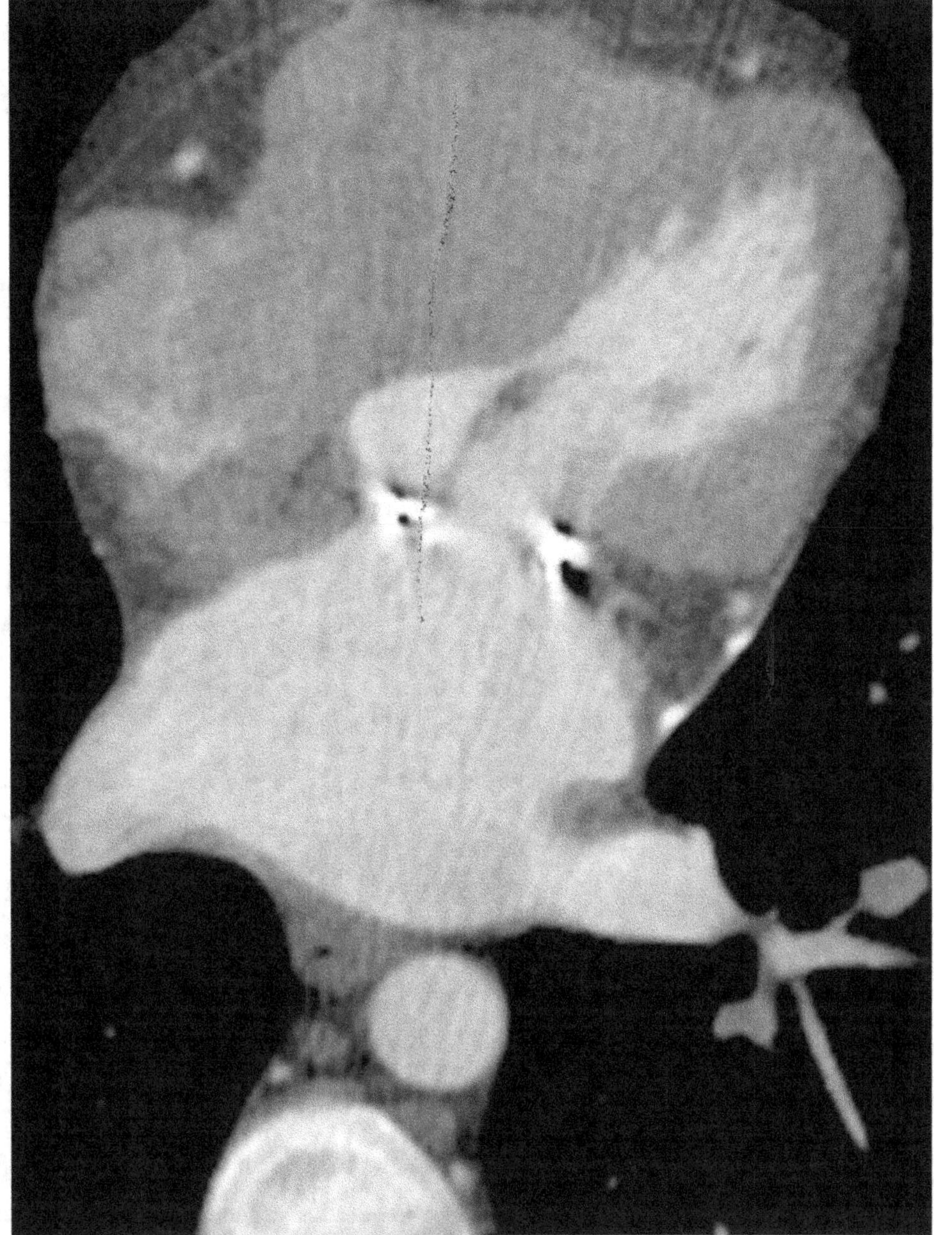

Figure 4. (Case #1) Computed tomographic image in the patient described. Shown here is the left atrium, the calcific deposits behind the mitral ring, and the left ventricular cavity. The orifice of the mitral valve is quite narrow. LA = left atrium; LV = left ventricle.

Disclosures

The authors have no conflicts of interest to disclose.

1. Roberts WC, Moore M, Ko JM, Hamman BL. Mitral valve replacement after failed mitral ring insertion with or without leaflet/chordal repair for pure mitral regurgitation. *Am J Cardiol* 2016;117:1790–1807.
2. Marwick TH, Stewart WJ, Currie PJ, Cosgrove DM. Mechanisms of failure of mitral valve repair: an echocardiographic study. *Am Heart J* 1991;122:149–156.
3. El Asmar B, Perier P, Couetil JP, Carpentier A. Failures in reconstructive mitral valve surgery. *J Med Liban* 1991;39:7–11.
4. Fernandez J, Joyce DH, Hirschfeld K, Chen C, Laub GW, Adkins MS, Anderson WA, Mackenzie JW, McGrath LB. Factors affecting mitral valve reoperation in 317 survivors after mitral valve reconstruction. *Ann Thorac Surg* 1992;54:440–448.
5. Niederhäuser U, Carrel T, von Segesser LK, Laske A, Turina M. Reoperation after mitral valve reconstruction: early and late results. *Eur J Cardiothorac Surg* 1993;7:34–37.
6. Cohn LH, Couper GS, Aranki SF, Rizzo RJ, Kinchla NM, Collins JJ Jr. Long-term results of mitral valve reconstruction for regurgitation of the myxomatous mitral valve. *J Thorac Cardiovasc Surg* 1994;107:143–151.
7. Carpentier AF, Lessana A, Relland JYM, Belli E, Mihaileanu S, Berrebi AJ, Palsky E, Loulmet DF. The "Physio-ring": an advanced concept in mitral valve annuloplasty. *Ann Thorac Surg* 1995;60:1177–1186.
8. Gillinov AM, Cosgrove DM, Lytle BW, Taylor PC, Stweart RW, McCarthy PM, Smedira NG, Muehrcke DD, Apperson-Hansen C, Loop FD. Reoperation for failure of mitral valve repair. *J Thorac Cardiovasc Surg* 1997;113:467–475.
9. David TE, Omran A, Armstrong S, Sun Z, Ivanov J. Long-term results of mitral valve repair for myxomatous disease with and without chordal

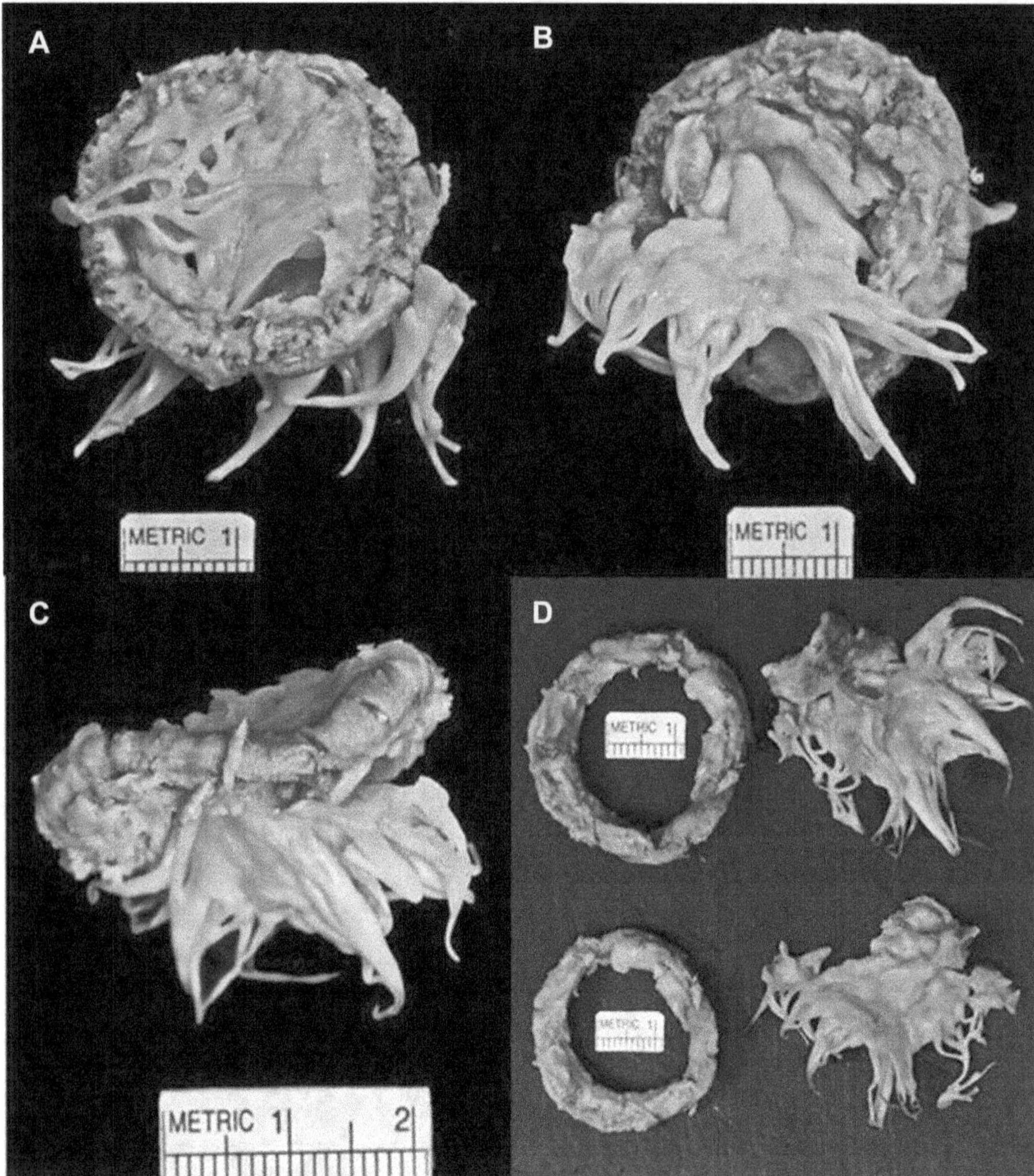

Figure 5. (Case #1) Shown here is the mitral valve with the circumferential ring attached *(A to C)* and after excision of the mitral valve from the circumferential ring *(D)*. *(A)* A view from what would be the left atrium showing the very small orifice of the mitral valve. *(B)* A view of the mitral valve within the mitral annular ring. *(C)* A side view of the mitral leaflets attached to the ring. *(D)* A view of the ring after detachment of the mitral valve. The top one shows the ring from what would be atrial side and the atrial aspect of the anterior mitral leaflet. A calcific fragment is attached to the anterior leaflet. The lower portion shows the ring from the ventricular aspect and the anterior mitral leaflet from the ventricular aspect.

replacement with expanded polytetrafluoroethylene sutures. *J Thorac Cardiovasc Surg* 1998;115:1279—1286.

10. Gillinov AM, Cosgrove DM, Blackstone EH, Diaz R, Arnold JH, Lytle BW, Smedira NG, Sabik JF, McCarthy PM, Loop FD. Durability of mitral valve repair for degenerative disease. *J Thorac Cardiovasc Surg* 1998;116:734—743.

11. Totaro P, Tulumello E, Fellini P, Rambaldini M, La Canna G, Coletti G, Zogno M, Lorusso R. Mitral valve repair for isolated prolapse of the anterior leaflet: an 11-year follow-up. *Eur J Cardiothorac Surg* 1999;15:119—126.

12. Smolens IA, Pagani FD, Deeb M, Prager RL, Sonnad SS, Bolling SF. Prophylactic mitral reconstruction for mitral regurgitation. *Ann Thorac Surg* 2001;72:1210—1216.

13. Braunberger E, Deloche A, Berrebi A, Fayssoil A, Celestin JA, Meimoun P, Chatellier G, Chauvaud S, Fabiani JN, Carpentier A. Very long-term results (more than 20 years) of valve repair with Carpentier's techniques in nonrheumatic mitral valve insufficiency. *Circulation* 2001;104:I8—I11.

14. Ibrahim MF, David TE. Mitral stenosis after mitral valve repair for non-rheumatic mitral regurgitation. *Ann Thorac Surg* 2002;73: 34—36.

15. David TE, Ivanov J, Armstrong S, Rakowski H. Late outcomes of mitral valve repair for floppy valves: implications for asymptomatic patients. *J Thorac Cardiovasc Surg* 2003;125:1143—1152.

16. David TE, Ivanov J, Armstrong S, Christie D, Rakowski H. A comparison of outcomes of mitral valve repair for degenerative disease with posterior, anterior, and bileaflet prolapse. *J Thorac Cardiovasc Surg* 2005;130:1242—1249.

17. Suri RM, Schaff HV, Dearani JA, Sundt TM III, Daly RC, Mullany CJ, Enriquez-Sarano M, Orszulak TA. Recurrent mitral regurgitation after

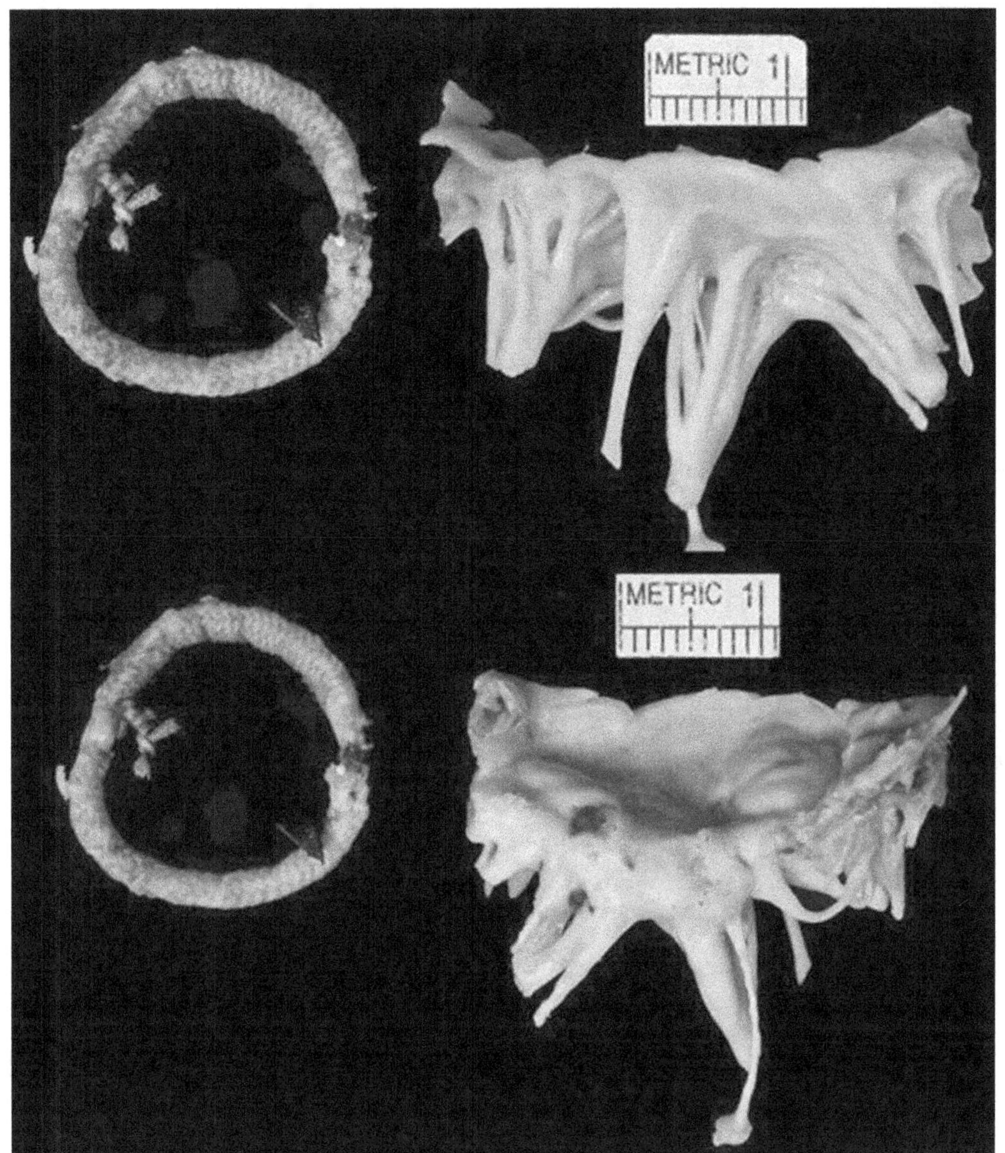

Figure 6. (Case #2) Operatively excised mitral ring *(left)* and anterior mitral leaflet *(right)* from the ventricular aspect *(upper)* and atrial aspect *(lower)*. The distal third of the leaflet is thickened by fibrous tissue and focal calcific deposits. Likewise, most chordae tendinae are thickened by fibrous tissue.

Table 2
Previously published reports describing frequency of mitral valve reoperation late for mitral stenosis after mitral valve repair for pure mitral regurgitation

Last Name of First Author (Year)	No. of Patients with MV Repair	MV Ring Inserted	Age at Original MV Repair (Years) Range (Mean)	Male: Female	Follow-up Time (Years) Range (Mean)	Reoperation	Interval between Operations (Years) Range (Mean)	MVR	No. developing MS following MV Repair	No. with MS having MVR
Asmar (1991)	1705	–	–	–	0-16 (_)	72 (4%)	0-13 (5.0±3.5)	61 (3%)	12 (0.7%)	12 (0.7%)
Fernandez (1992)	313	4 (1%)	9-81 (57)	110:203	1-20 (7)	63 (20%)	1-15 (6)	–	8 (3%)	–
Niederhäuser (1993)	346	5 (1%)	_ - _ (47±16)	–	_ - _ (5)	68 (20%)	_ - _ (7)	62 (18%)	17 (5%)	17 (5%)
Ibrahim (2002)	478	405 (85%)	51-61 (56)	–	1-11 (4.1±2.8)	–	4-9 (6)	3 (0.6%)	4 (0.8%)	3 (0.6%)
David (2003)	488	488 (100%)	_ - _ (58±13)	347:71	3-19 (7)	22 (5%)	_ - _ (_)	18 (4%)	2 (0.4%)	2 (0.4%)
David (2005)	701	668 (95%)	18-88 (58±13)	512:189	0-23 (6.9±4.0)	27 (4%)	5-8 (_)	–	3 (0.4%)	–
Suri (2006)	145	–	_ - _ (66±12)	102:43	_ - _ (3.3±4.1)	145 (100%)	_ - _ (4.1±5.1)	81 (56%)	1 (1%)	0
Chung (2007)	294	294 (100%)	_ - _ (53±13)	175:119	(3.0±1.9)	7 (2%)	(1-7) (_)	–	14 (5%)	3 (1%)
Chan (2016)	829	829 (100%)	_ - _ (64±13)	567:262	_ - _ (4.3±3.5)	21 (3%)	_ - _ (8.2)	14 (2%)	3 (0.4%)	0
Lazam (2017)	1709	–	_ - _ (65±12)	1265:444	4-18 (9)	95 (5%)	–	–	4 (0.2%)	–

MS = mitral stenosis; MV = mitral valve; MVR = mitral valve replacement; – = no information available.

Table 3

Previously published case reports describing the late development of mitral stenosis following mitral valve repair

Last Name of First Author (year)	Sex	Age at repair (years)	Cause of the MR	Quadrangular Resection of PML	Duran Ring Inserted (Size: mm)	Interval between repair and presentation of mitral stenosis (years)	Mitral valve area (cm^2)	Mean mitral valve gradient by echocardiogram (mmHg)	MVR	Interval between initial repair and MVR or PBMV or second operation (years)
Tanaka (2003)	Woman	50	MVP	+	+ (25)	3	–	–	+	3
Nishida (2005)	Woman	43	MVP	+	+ (27)	3	0.67[*]	22	+	4
Song (2010)	Woman	57	MVP	+	+ (25)	7	–	10	0[§]	7
Sachpekidis (2012)	Man	60	IC	0	+ (27)	5	1.29	10	0[‡]	–[†]
Salenger (2016)	Woman	22	IC	0	+ (25)	12	0.6	28	0[§]	12

IC = ischemic cardiomyopathy; MR = mitral regurgitation; MVP = mitral valve prolapse; MVR = mitral valve replacement; PBMV = percutaneous balloon mitral valvuloplasty; PML = posterior mitral leaflet.

[*] At cardiac catheterization.

[†] At the second operation the ring and pannus tissue were excised and a commissurotomy was performed.

[‡] Refused operation.

[§] The patient underwent PBMV.

repair: should the mitral valve be re-repaired? *J Thorac Cardiovasc Surg* 2006;132:1390–1397.

18. De Bonis M, Lorusso R, Lapenna E, Kassem S, De Cicco G, Torracca L, Maisano F, La Canna G, Alfieri O. Similar long-term results of mitral valve repair for anterior compared with posterior leaflet prolapse. *J Thorac Cardiovasc Surg* 2006;131:364–370.

19. Suri RM, Schaff HV, Dearani JA, Sundt TM III, Daly RC, Mullany CJ, Enriquez-Sarano M, Orszulak TA. Survival advantage and improved durability of mitral repair for leaflet prolapse subsets in the current era. *Ann Thorac Surg* 2006;82:819–827.

20. Dumont E, Gillinov AM, Blackstone EH, Sabik JF III, Svensson LG, Mihaljevic T, Houghtaling PL, Lytle BW. Reoperation after mitral valve repair for degenerative disease. *Ann Thorac Surg* 2007;84:444–450.

21. Chung CH, Kim JB, Choo SJ, Kim KS, Song H, Song MG, Song JK, Kang DH, Lee JW. Long-term outcomes after mitral ring annuloplasty for degenerative mitral regurgitation: Duran ring versus Carpentier-Edwards ring. *J Heart Valve Dis* 2007;16:536–545.

22. Chan V, Elmistekawy E, Ruel M, Hynes M, Mesana TG. How does mitral valve repair fail in patients with prolapse?-Insights from longitudinal echocardiographic follow-up. *Ann Thorac Surg* 2016;102:1459–1465.

23. Lazam S, Vanoverschelde JL, Tribouilloy C, Grigioni F, Suri RM, Avierinos JF, de Meester C, Barbieri A, Rusinaru D, Russo A, Pasquet A, Michelena HI, Huebner M, Maalouf J, Clavel MA, Szymanski C, Enriquez-Sarano M. Twenty-year outcome after mitral repair versus replacement for severe degenerative mitral regurgitation: analysis of a large, prospective, multicenter, international registry. *Circulation* 2017;135:410–422.

24. Tanaka K, Makuuchi H, Naruse Y, Kobayashi T, Havashi I, Takayama T, Namifusa Y. Mitral stenosis due to fibrous tissue overgrowth after mitral valve repair. *J Cardiovasc Surg* 2003;44:59–60.

25. Nishida H, Takahara Y, Takeuchi S, Mogi K. Mitral stenosis after mitral valve repair using the Duran flexible annuloplasty ring for degenerative mitral regurgitation. *J Heart Valve Dis* 2005;14:563–564.

26. Song S, Cho SH, Yang JH, Park PW. Repair for mitral stenosis due to pannus formation after Duran ring annuloplasty. *Ann Thorac Surg* 2010;90:93–94.

27. Sachpekidis V, Agatziotis M, Styliadis I, Mosialos L, Kaprinis I, Monaghan MJ, Adamopoulos C. Three-dimensional imaging of pannus overgrowth after mitral valve repair. *Echocardiography* 2012;29:210–213.

28. Salenger R, Diao X, Dawood MY, Herr DL, Sample GA, Pichard A, Gammie JS. Percutaneous rescue for critical mitral stenosis late after mitral valve repair. *Ann Thorac Surg* 2016;102:417–418.

Hazards of Mitral Valve Replacement for Mitral Stenosis Caused by Massive Mitral Annular Calcium With or Without Aortic Valve Replacement for Aortic Stenosis

William C. Roberts, MD*

Mitral annular calcium (MAC) is common in older adults in the Western World and if extensive may cause mitral stenosis . The purpose of this report is to describe outcomes of 12 patients having mitral valve replacement for mitral stenosis secondary to massive MAC. Operatively excised deposits of calcium removed from the mitral annular area and the accompanying stenotic mitral valves were examined and then the patients' medical records were examined to confirm the diagnosis and the degree of valvular dysfunction. A total of 12 patients with massive MAC causing mitral stenosis and receiving mitral valve replacement with or without aortic valve replacement for aortic stenosis were observed in 2013 to 2015. Of the 12 patients, 7 died from 5 to 44 days (mean 19) after the valve operation and all had "stormy" postoperative courses; one survived 150 days and another, 600 days; the remaining 3 were improved by the operation and are alive 22, 27, and 59 months postoperatively. In conclusion, the high mortality in these patients suggests that mitral valve replacement in the setting of massive MAC be considered with caution.   © 2018 Elsevier Inc. All rights reserved. (Am J Cardiol 2019;123:650−657)

Deposits of calcium beneath the posterior mitral leaflet and especially near its attachment to the left atrial and left ventricular junctional regions, so called *mitral annular calcium* (MAC), is relatively common in older patients, especially in women, in patients with chronic renal disease, in those with left ventricular outflow obstruction (aortic stenosis [AS] and hypertrophic cardiomyopathy), and in younger persons with mitral valve prolapse, mucopolysaccharidosis and the Marfan syndrome.[1−8] In older patients MAC is usually accompanied by calcific deposits in the epicardial coronary arteries and in the aortic valve cusps, producing what has been termed "the senile cardiac calcification syndrome"[9] (Figure 1). The quantity of calcium in the mitral annular region varies from minimal to massive and when the latter is the case the result may be mitral stenosis (MS), especially in the setting of associated AS.[10−15] We have encountered through the years many patients who have had aortic valve replacement for AS and who had massive MAC but no operative procedure was carried out on the mitral valve (Figure 2). In recent times in patients with combined AS and massive MAC causing MS there has been a tendency among some surgeons to replace the mitral valve as well as the aortic valve in this scenario.[16−25] This report describes certain clinical and morphologic findings in 12 patients with massive MAC causing MS and leading to isolated mitral valve replacement or to combined mitral and aortic valve replacement, the latter for AS.

Methods

Since March 1993, I have examined, described, and submitted the report on all surgical specimens excised from the heart or aorta at Baylor University Medical Center (BUMC). During a recent 3-year period—2013, 2014, and 2015—portions of the mitral valve in 130 patients were submitted to the surgical pathology unit of the department of pathology at BUMC (Figure 3). Of the 130 patients, 58 (45%) had mitral valve repair for pure mitral regurgitation (no element of stenosis), and 73 (56%) had mitral valve replacement. Of the latter 72 patients, 53 (74%) had isolated mitral valve replacement (only the mitral valve was replaced) and 19 (26%) had replacement of both the mitral and aortic valves. Of the 53 patients with isolated mitral valve replacement; 16 (30%) had mitral stenosis resulting from massive MAC in 6 and from rheumatic heart disease in 10. Of the 19 patients having combined mitral and aortic valve replacements, 10 had combined mitral stenosis and aortic stenosis, the result of rheumatic heart disease, and in 6 from massive MAC. This report focuses on the 6 patients having MS and isolated mitral replacement from massive MAC, and on the 4 patients who had both mitral and aortic valve replacement for combined MS resulting from massive MAC and aortic valve stenosis. Additionally, 2 other patients with massive MAC causing MS and associated with AS and operated on at another Dallas hospital also were included in this study.

The medical records in all of the 130 patients were examined.

Departments of Internal Medicine (Division of Cardiology) and Pathology, and the Baylor Scott & White Heart and Vascular Institute, Baylor University Medical Center, a part of Baylor Scott & White Health, Dallas, Texas. Manuscript received October 3, 2018; revised manuscript received November 12, 2018; revised manuscript received and accepted November 12, 2018.

See page 656 for disclosure information.

*Corresponding author: Tel: (214) 820-7911; fax: (214) 820-7533.

E-mail address: william.roberts1@bswhealth.org

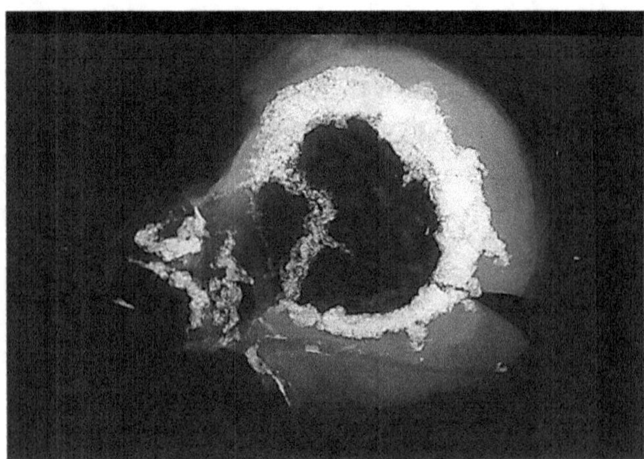

Figure 1. Shown here is a radiograph of the heart specimen at autopsy in an 82-year-old woman who died of volvulus of the colon. She never had symptoms of cardiac dysfunction. The amount of calcium in the mitral annular area is enormous. The calcium behind posterior mitral leaflet forms a beautiful "C" and the bar of calcium below the aortic valve is that on the ventricular aspect of anterior leaflet. Calcific deposits also are present in each of the three valve cusps causing some degree of aortic stenosis. Additionally, calcium is present focally in the left circumflex and left anterior descending coronary arteries. (Figure reproduced from Roberts WC, Perloff JK. Mitral valvular disease: A clinicopathologic survey of the conditions causing the mitral valve to function abnormally. *Ann Intern Med* 1972 Dec; 77:939–975.)

"Massive MAC" was defined by the presence of a huge quantity of calcium underlying the posterior mitral leaflet forming a circle C and extending across all or nearly all of the ventricular aspect of the anterior mitral leaflet to "close" the "C" forming a circle O. Examples of massive MAC forming a circle O are shown in Figures 1 and 2.

The present study includes all patients having mitral valve replacement for massive MAC encountered at BUMC during the 3-year period (2013 to 2015). Several other patients having mitral valve replacement for mitral valve prolapse causing mitral regurgitation had small focal deposits of calcium behind posterior mitral leaflet but in no patients were the deposits behind mitral leaflet large and in none did calcium extend across the ventricular aspect of anterior mitral leaflet.

Results

Pertinent clinical and morphologic data in these 12 patients were sought and the findings are summarized in Table 1. The 12 patients ranged in age from 25 to 82 years (median 59); 8 were women and 4 were men. Six patients had isolated mitral valve replacement and 6 had combined mitral and aortic valve replacement.

Preoperatively, the peak systolic pulmonary pressures ranged from 50 to 117 mm Hg (average 79); the pulmonary artery wedge-left ventricular mean diastolic gradients at rest ranged from 6 to 23 mm Hg (average 11) and the peak systolic left ventricular to systemic artery peak pressure gradients ranged from 20 to 28 mm Hg. Four patients had considerable coronary arterial narrowing by angiogram, 3 of whom had coronary bypass performed. Preoperatively,

8 patients had atrial fibrillation, 1 had complete heart block, and 1 had right bundle branch block. Six patients had diabetes mellitus. The body mass index (11 patients) ranged from 21 to 52 kg/m^2 including 8 patients (73%) in whom the value was $\geq$30 kg/m^2. The 12 patients were operated on by 5 different surgeons.

Of the 12 patients, 7 died from 5 to 44 days after valve replacement, 1 at 150 days and 1 other at 600 days after the valve replacement. The remaining 3 were improved by the operation and are alive 22, 27, and 59 months after the valve operation. The operatively-excised mitral specimens ranged in weight from 1.92 to 7.20 g. The operatively excised aortic valves (3 patients) weighed 0.49, 1.20, and 2.95 g, respectively.

Several of the operatively excised mitral and aortic specimens are illustrated in Figures 4 to 8. Autopsies were performed in 2 patients: in each considerable quantities of calcium remained in the mitral annular area. Periannular mitral disruptions were present in each of the 2 autopsied patients.

Discussion

It is apparent from study of these hitherto described 12 patients that mitral valve replacement in the setting of *massive* MAC is hazardous. Nine of the 12 patients have died, 7 within 45 days of the operation and 2 others 150 and 600 days, respectively, postoperatively. The postoperative courses in the 7 early deaths were complicated by stroke; excessive bleeding (requiring return to the operating room); parabasilar mitral regurgitation; long periods of intubation, and usually evidence of inadequate cardiac output ("multiorgan failure").

In the early days of cardiac valve replacement (1960s and 1970s), combined mitral and aortic valve replacement was a frequent procedure and was usually because of rheumatic heart disease, most commonly resulting in stenosis of both valves, occasionally causing pure regurgitation of both valves, and rarely producing 1 stenotic and 1 purely regurgitant valve. Today in the Western World, rheumatic heart disease, of course, is far less frequent than in the past, and now both isolated MS and that combined with AS may commonly be the result of massive MAC. Replacement of both left-sided cardiac valves at the same operation is a formidable operation, especially when both valves are stenotic.[26] In this latter setting, usually the left ventricular free wall is thickened, the left ventricular cavity is not dilated, and the ascending aorta is not dilated. When the mitral dysfunction is caused by massive MAC the operation is even more formidable. At least in the patients with combined rheumatic MS and AS the patients are usually relatively young, and the mitral annulus is not calcified. In the patients with MAC of sufficient quantity to obstruct the mitral orifice, the patients are usually in the older age group.

The Tiron E. David group[16,18] in Toronto has written extensively on methods and results for replacing and/or repairing the mitral valve in the setting of "extensive" MAC. In one of their reports the operative mortality was 6.2 times that occurring in patients having mitral valve

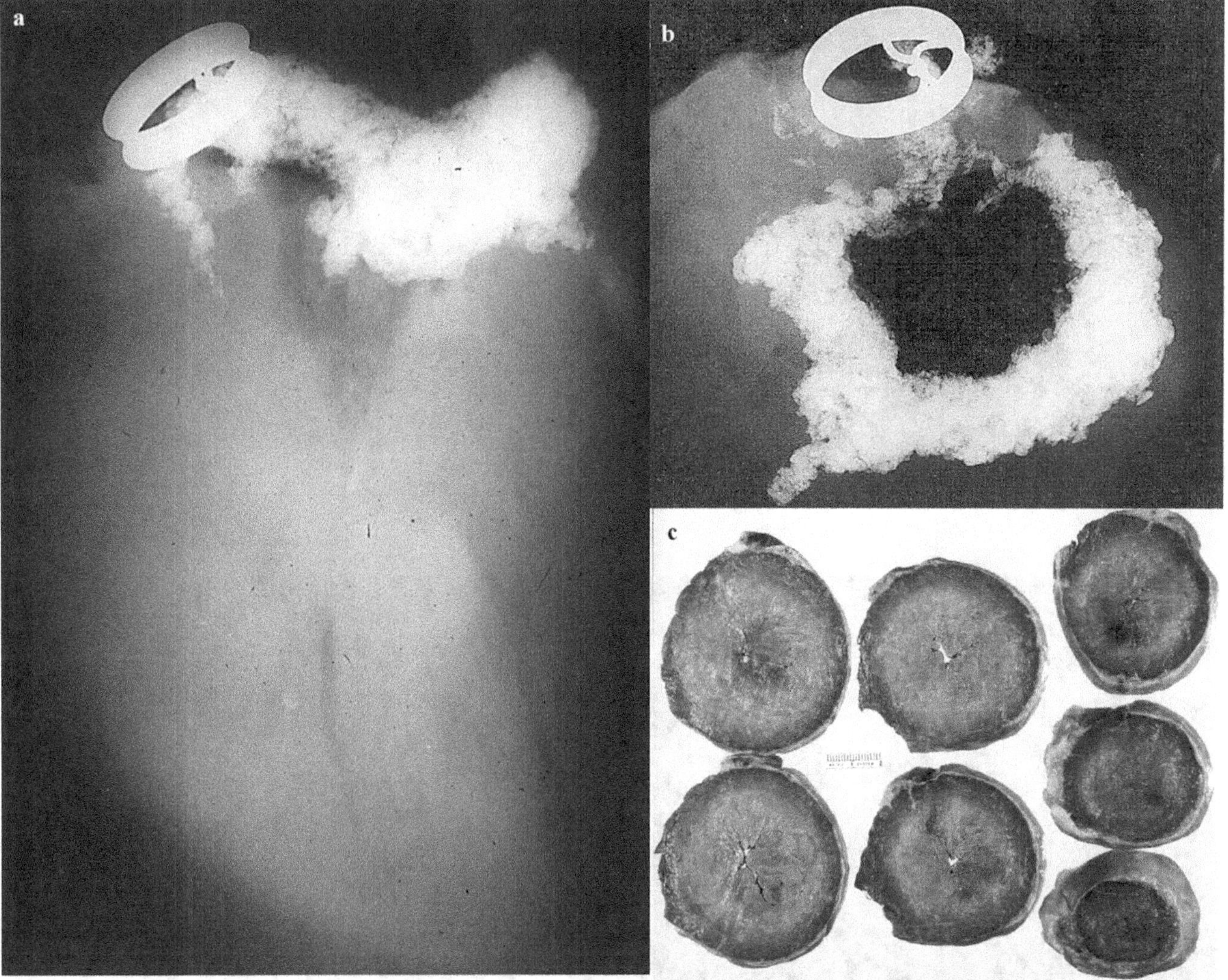

Figure 2. Shown here in *a*, *b*, and *c* views are radiographs of the heart at necropsy. There is massive mitral annular calcium which forms nearly a "C" as shown in *b*. The aortic valve was replaced with a Bjork-Shailey prosthesis. No replacement of the mitral valve was attempted even though the mitral orifice was stenotic. *c* shows transverse sections of the left ventricle to illustrate its small cavity. Death occurs in peak systole, so the left ventricular cavity would be larger during ventricular diastole.

procedures at their institution without MAC. Early postoperative complications in their 54 MAC patients included re-exploration for bleeding (9%), permanent heart block requiring a pacemaker (20%), reoperation later related to valve complications (7%), late postoperative thromboembolic events (9%), and late major hemorrhagic complications (5%). Their series of 54 patients having mitral operations—combined with aortic valve replacement for AS in 23 (43%)—appear to be the best from anywhere in the setting of extensive MAC. Possibly, most of their patients had smaller quantities of MAC than the patients described herein. In 31 (57%) of their 54 patients the MAC was located only behind the posterior mitral leaflet and did not extend across the ventricular aspect of anterior mitral leaflet as it did in the 12 patients described herein. These investigators emphasize the difficulty of the operation and state the following:

"Extensive calcification of the mitral annulus may present a formidable surgical challenge during mitral valve surgery. The patient is at risk from such potentially fatal complications as intractable hemorrhage, atrioventricular disruption, and ventricular rupture...Although we recommend removal of the calcium bar, this is a major undertaking and should not be considered lightly..."

Another unemphasized difficulty of mitral replacement in the setting of massive MAC and associated AS is the lack of dilatation of the left ventricular cavity in most of these patients including all 12 described herein.[26] Shown in Figure 2 is the heart of a 70-year-old woman who died shortly after replacement of a severely stenotic congenitally bicuspid aortic valve (peak transvalvular gradient = 153 mm Hg). A 15-mm Hg mean diastolic pressure gradient was present between left atrium

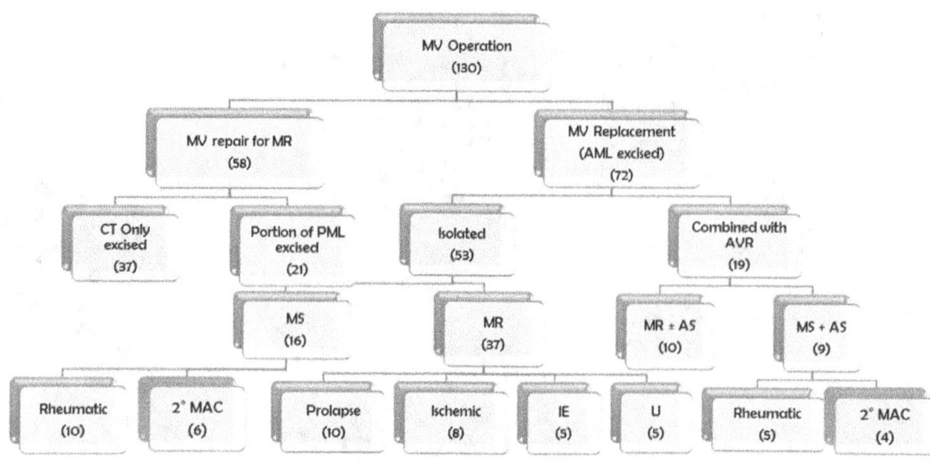

Figure 3. Reason for mitral valve operations at Baylor University Medical Center at Dallas during the 3 years: 2013, 2014, and 2015. Abbreviations: AML = anterior mitral leaflet; AS = aortic stenosis; AVR = aortic valve replacement; CT = chordae tendineae; IE = infective endocarditis; MAC = mitral annular calcium; MR = mitral regurgitation; MV = mitral valve; PML = posterior mitral leaflet; U = unknown.

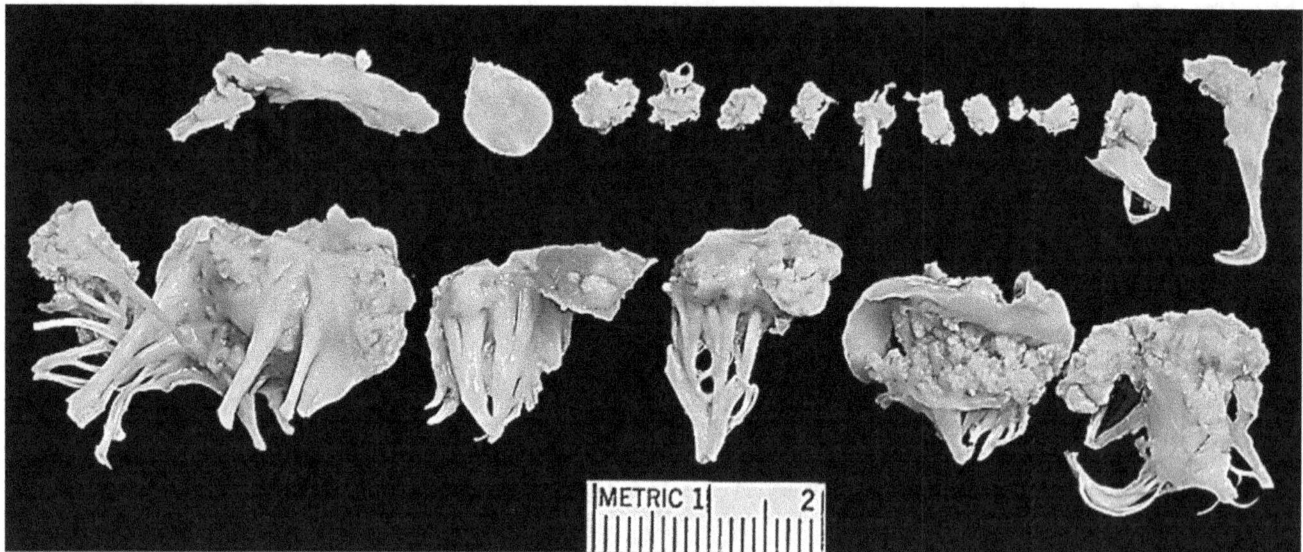

Figure 4. Case #1, Table 1. Portions of the posterior and anterior leaflets of the mitral valve and fragments of calcium excised from the mitral annular region. Calcium extends across the ventricular aspect of the anterior mitral leaflet.

and left ventricle. The mitral valve, however, was not replaced. The reason for showing these photos is to emphasize the small size of the left ventricular cavity in the setting of combined MS and AS. The small sized ventricular cavity makes it especially difficult to insert a prosthesis or a bioprosthesis in the mitral position in addition to the difficulty in excising the massive MAC in this scenario.

There has been recent interest in transcatheter mitral valve implantation in patients with MS caused by MAC.[27,28] Sud and colleagues[27] reviewed 10 previously-reported case studies of patients having transcatheter mitral valve implantation and 44 patients in a global registry having the percutaneous procedure. In the individual case studies, no deaths were reported. In the series of 44 patients, the 1-year all-cause mortality was 36%. The transvalvular gradients were reduced in most patients although nonfatal complications were frequent. Guerrero and associates[28] updated the MAC Global Registry multicenter data to include 106 patients followed >1 year. One and 12-month all-cause mortality was 25% and 54%, respectively. Of the 77 patients who were alive 30 days after the procedure, 49 (64%) were alive at 1 year. The mean transmitral pressure gradient by echocardiogram, available in 34 patients, at 1 year was 6±2 mm Hg. Examination of hearts with massive MAC causing MS as shown in Figures 1 and 2 suggest why both the surgical and the percutaneous approach for treatment of MS secondary to massive MAC is fraught with difficulty.

One of the reviewers of this manuscript asked why the results of the present study were so much worse than those described by Ng and colleagues[20] in 2000. Study of the Na report suggests that their 37 patients had far less mitral annular calcium than the patients described herein. None of Ng's

Table 1
Pertinent findings in the 12 patients with massive mitral annular calcium and mitral valve replacement for mitral stenosis with or without aortic valve replacement for aortic stenosis

Case	Age (years)	Sex	MS	MVR	Mitral valve weight (g)	Substitute mitral valve (mm)	AS	AVR	Aortic valve weight (g)	Substitute aortic valve (mm)	CKD	Narrowed coronary arteries	AF	BMI (Kg/m²)	DM	Interval VR →D (days)
1	39	F	+	+	6.0	SJM (25)	0	0	—	—	+(H)	0	0	21	0	8
2	52	F	+	+	3.9	Bioprosthesis (29)	0	0	—	—	0	0	0	40	+	Alive [†]
3	58	M	+	+	3.2	Bioprosthesis (27)	0	0	—	—	+ (RT)	+ (CABG)	0	30	+	Alive [‡]
4	61	F	+	+	1.5	SJM (33)	0	0	—	—	0	0	+	38	0	Alive [§]
5	62	F	+	+	5.7	SJM (27)	0	0	—	—	0	0	+	28	0	5
6	76	M	+	+	1.9	Bicor (29)	0	0	—	—	0	+ (CABG)	+	36	+	44
7	40	M	+	+	3.3	$O_2 - X$ (25)	+ [*]	+	3.0	Carbomedius (21)	+(P)	0	+	34	0	600
8	42	F	+	+	1.9	SJM (27)	+	+ [†]	—	SJM (21)	+(H)	0	+	—	0	150
9	71	F	+	+	—	St. Jude Epic (←)	+	+	—	Magna Ease (21)	0	+ (CABG)	+	31	+	32
10	74	F	+	+	7.2	ATS Mech (24)	+	+	1.2	ATS Mech (20)	+	0	+	36	+	12
11	76	F	+	+	4.7	Bicor (25)	+	+	0.5	CE (19)	+	0	0	52	+	25
12	82	M	+	+	—	Edwards Magna (27)	+	+	—	—	0	+	+	—	0	11

Abbreviations: AF = atrial fibrillation; AS = aortic stenosis; AVR = aortic valve replacement; BMI = body mass index; CABG = coronary artery bypass grafting; CKD = chronic kidney disease; D = death; DM = diabetes mellitus; F = female; H = hemodialysis initiated months or years before MVR; LV = left ventricle; M = male; MS = mitral stenosis; MVR = mitral valve replacement; P = peritoneal dialysis; RT = renal transplant earlier; VR = valve replacement.

[*] BAV;

[†] AVR 22 months before excision of the bioprosthesis in the aortic valve position and replacement of the MV;

[‡] Alive 36 months postoperatively. Improved, less breathlessness, twenty pounds less (250→230);

[§] Alive 59 months postoperatively. Much improved. Little breathlessness;

[¶] Alive 27 months postoperatively. Greatly improved. Nearly no breathlessness. Thirty pounds weight loss (240→210).

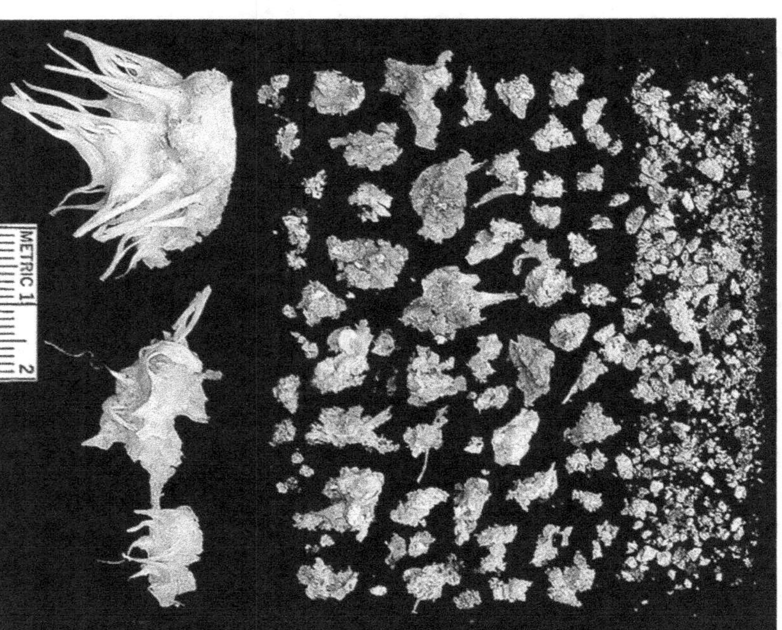

Figure 5. Case 5, Table 1. Shown here are large deposits of calcium excised from the mitral annular region and the anterior mitral leaflet with a bar of calcium across its ventricular aspect and two fragments of posterior leaflet. The quantity of calcium in the mitral annular area was obviously enormous.

patients had mitral stenosis, only mitral regurgitation and it is likely that much heavier deposits of calcium are required to obstruct the mitral orifice by annular calcium than to produce only regurgitation. It is unlikely that the annular calcium behind posterior leaflet extended across the ventricular surface of anterior mitral leaflet in Ng's patients as it did in the patients described herein. Indeed Ng et al wrote: "Five patients were excluded from (their) study due to severe calcification of nearly the entire annulus..." None of Ng's patients had associated aortic stenosis, a feature in half of the patients in the present study and something that tends to make the left ventricular cavity smaller and probably the mitral orifice smaller. Finally, none of Ng's patients had mitral valve replacement as did all the patients in the present study.

The mechanism of development of MAC and its commonly associated AS is not entirely clear but most likely is a consequence of atherosclerosis, although that word would have to be redefined to include MAC and AS under that heading. Most young people living in the Western World have yellow deposits on the undersurface of the posterior mitral leaflet and fewer such deposits on the ventricular surface of anterior mitral leaflet. Additionally, similar deposits occur on the aortic aspects of the aortic valve cusps, whether its structure is tricuspid or bicuspid. In later life the lipid deposits may transform into calcific deposits, and, depending on the quantity of those deposits in the 2 valves, may or may not

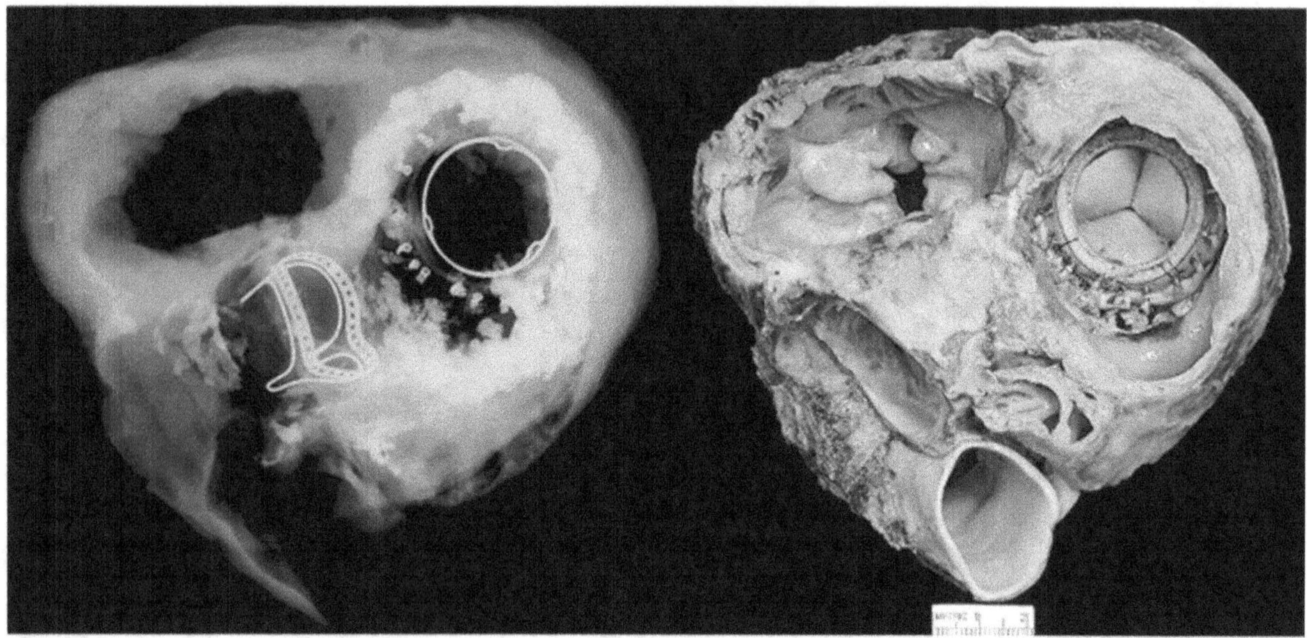

Figure 6. Case #9, Table 1. Shown here is a radiograph of the heart specimen at necropsy on the *left* and the actual specimen shown on the *right*. Both the mitral and aortic valves were replaced because of stenosis. A large amount of calcium was removed from the mitral annular region at operation but there is still a great deal of calcium left in that area. The more anterolateral portion of the mitral annulus had a communication between the cloth ring and the annulus so there was a para-annular leak. Heavy calcific deposits are also seen in the epicardial coronary arteries.

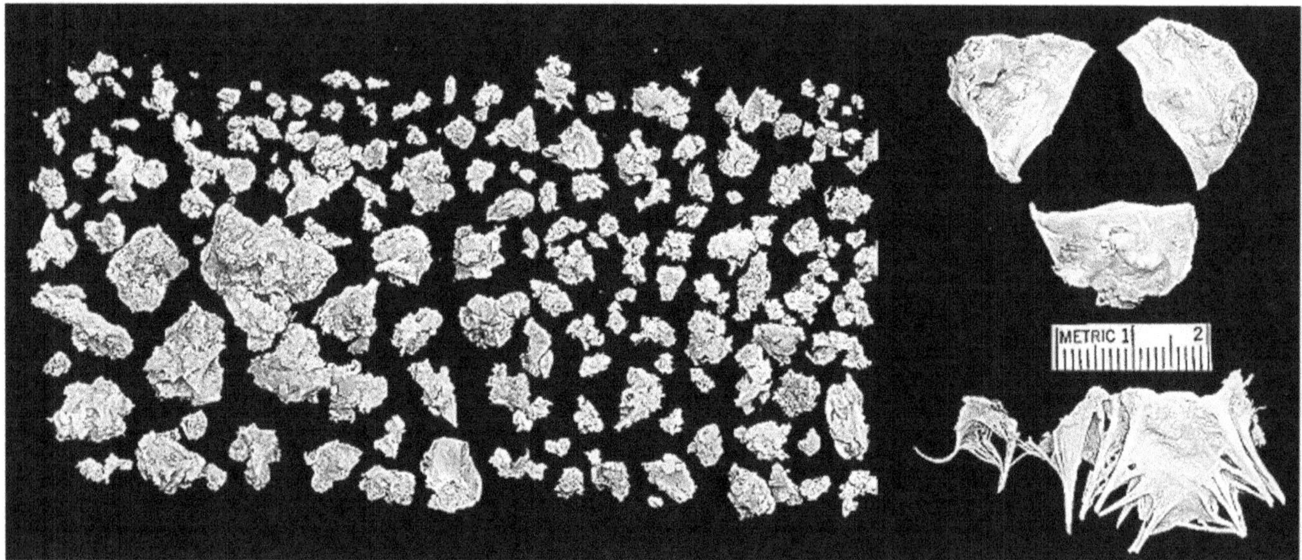

Figure 7. Case 10, Table 1. Shown here are huge calcific fragments excised from the mitral annular region (*left*), the operatively excised aortic valve cusps containing calcific fragments (*top right*), and the ventricular aspect of anterior mitral leaflet (*bottom right*). About half of the anterior leaflet has a bar of calcium extending across its ventricular aspect.

lead to symptoms of cardiac dysfunction. Because "atherosclerosis" preferentially affects the systemic arteries, associated coronary narrowing in these patients is common.

In conclusion, performing mitral valve replacement in the setting of *massive* MAC is both difficult and hazardous, even more so when the aortic valve is also stenotic.

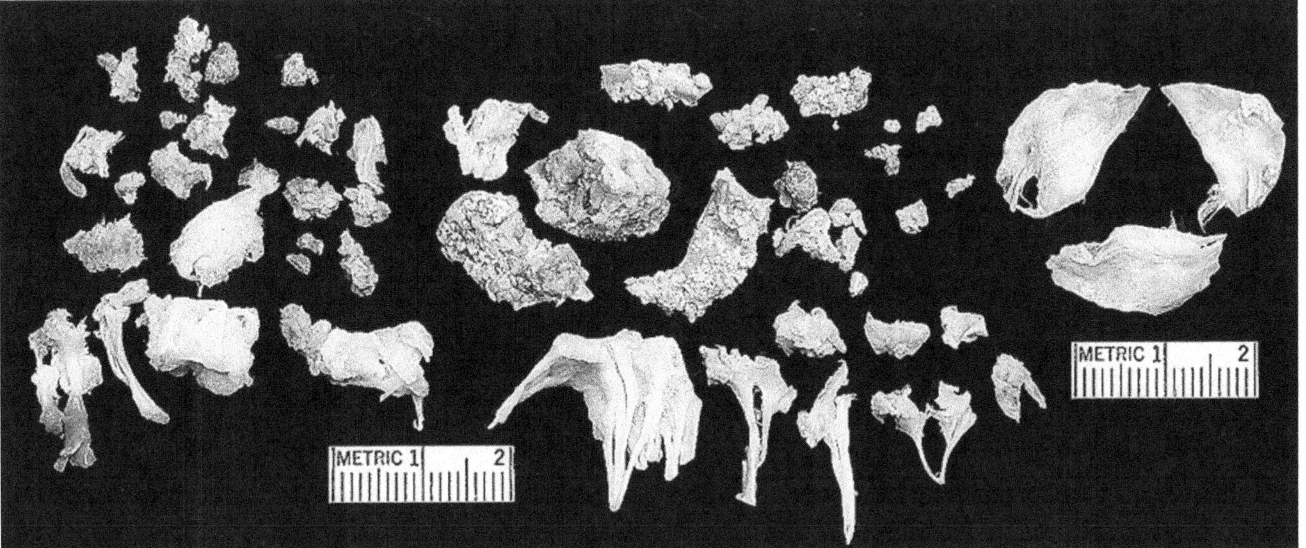

Figure 8. Case 11, Table 1. Shown here is both the operatively excised mitral valve and the 3-cuspid aortic valve plus the numerous calcific fragments excised from the mitral annular region. These fragments together weighed 4.72 g. Of course, not all the calcium in the mitral annular region was excised.

Disclosures

The author has no conflict of interests to disclose.

1. Korn D, DeSanctis RW, Sell S. Massive calcification of the mitral annulus. A clinicopathological study of fourteen cases. *N Engl J Med* 1962;267:900–908.
2. Roberts WC, Shirani J. Comparison of cardiac findings at necropsy in octogenarians, nonagenarians, and centenarians. *Am J Cardiol* 1998;82:627–631.
3. Roberts WC, Taylor MA, Shirani J. Cardiac findings at necropsy in patients with chronic kidney disease maintained on chronic hemodialysis. *Medicine* 2012;91:165–178.
4. Roberts WC, Vowels TJ, Filardo G, Ko JM, Mathur RP, Shirani J. Natural history of unoperated aortic stenosis during a 50-year period of cardiac valve replacement. *Am J Cardiol* 2013;112:541–553.
5. Motamed HE, Roberts WC. Frequency and significance of mitral annular calcium in hypertrophic cardiomyopathy: analysis of 200 necropsy patients. *Am J Cardiol* 1987;60:877–884.
6. Roberts WC, McIntosh CL, Wallace RB. Mechanisms of severe mitral regurgitation in mitral valve prolapse determined from analysis of operatively excised valves. *Am Heart J* 1987;113:1316–1323.
7. Renteria VG, Ferrans VJ, Roberts WC. The heart in the Hurler Syndrome: gross, histologic and ultrastructural observations in five necropsy cases. *Am J Cardiol* 1976;38:487–501.
8. Roberts WC. Morphologic aspects of cardiac valve dysfunction. *Am Heart J* 1992;123:1610–1632.
9. Roberts WC. The senile cardiac calcification syndrome. *Am J Cardiol* 1986;58:572–574.
10. Roberts WC, Waller BF. Mitral valve "anular" calcium forming a complete circle of "O" configuration: clinical and necropsy observations. *Am Heart J* 1981;101:619–621.
11. Theleman KP, Grayburn PA, Roberts WC. Mitral "annular" calcium forming a complete circle "O" causing mitral stenosis in association with a stenotic congenitally bicuspid aortic valve and severe coronary artery disease. *Am J Geriatr Cardiol* 2006;15:58–61.
12. Hammer WJ, Roberts WC, deLeon AC Jr. "Mitral stenosis" secondary to combined "massive" mitral annular calcific deposits and small, hypertrophied left ventricles: hemodynamic documentation in four patients. *Am J Med* 1978;64:371–376.
13. Ramirez J, Flowers NC. Severe mitral stenosis secondary to massive calcification of the mitral annulus with unusual echocardiographic manifestations. *Clin Cardiol* 1980;3:284–287.
14. Osterberger LE, Goldstein S, Khaja F, Lakier JB. Functional mitral stenosis in patients with massive mitral annular calcification. *Circulation* 1981;64:472–476.
15. Pressman GS, Agarwal A, Braitman LE, Muddassir SM. Mitral annular calcium causing mitral stenosis. *Am J Cardiol* 2010;105:389–391.
16. David TE, Feindel CM, Armstrong S, Sun Z. Reconstruction of the mitral annulus: a ten-year experience. *J Thorac Cardiovasc Surg* 1995;110:1323–1332.
17. Carpenter AF, Pellerin M, Fuzellier JF, Relland JYM. Extensive calcification of the mitral valve annulus: pathology and surgical management. *J Thorac Cardiovasc Surg* 1996;111:718–729.
18. David TE, Kuo J, Armstrong S. Aortic and mitral valve replacement with reconstruction of the intervalvular fibrous body. *J Thorac Cardiovasc Surg* 1997;114:766–772.
19. Lin PY, Kan CD, Luo CY, Yang YJ. Mitral valve replacement in the presence of massive posterior annular calcification. *J Card Surg* 1999;14:266–269.
20. Ng CK, Punzengruber C, Pachinger O, Nesser J, Auer H, Franke H, Hartl P. Valve repair in mitral regurgitation complicated by severe annulus calcification. *Ann Thorac Surg* 2000;70:53–58.
21. Fasol R, Mahdjoobian K, Joubert-Hubner E. Mitral repair in patients with severely calcified annulus: feasibility, surgery and results. *J Heart Valve Dis* 2002;11:153–159.
22. Feindel CM, Tufail Z, David TE, Ivanov J, Armstrong S. Mitral valve surgery in patients with extensive calcification of the mitral annulus. *J Thorac Cardiovasc Surg* 2003;126:777–782.
23. DiStefano S, Lopez J, Flórez S, Rey J, Arevalo A, San Román A. Building a new annulus: a technique for mitral valve replacement in heavily calcified annulus. *Ann Thorac Surg* 2009;87:1625–1627.
24. Atoui R, Lash V, Mohammadi S, Cecere R. Intra-atrial implantation of a mitral valve prosthesis in a heavily calcified mitral annulus. *Eur J Cardiothorac Surg* 2009;36:776-768.
25. Nomura A, Fukuda I, Daitoku K, Fukui K. Enucleation of calcium core and in-situ valve replacement for massive posterior mitral annular calcification. *Interact Cardiovasc Thorac Surg* 2011;12:652–654.
26. Roberts WC, Sullivan MF. Clinical and necropsy observations early after simultaneous replacement of the mitral and aortic valves. *Am J Cardiol* 1986;58:1067–1084.
27. Sud K, Agarwal S, Parashar A, Raza MQ, Patel K, Min D, Rodriguez LL, Krishnaswamy A, Mick SL, Gillinov AM, Tuzcu M, Kapadia SR. Degenerative mitral stenosis: unmet need for percutaneous interventions. *Circulation* 2016;133:1594–1604.
28. Guerrero M, Urena M, Himbert D, Wang DD4, Eleid M5, Kodali S, George I, Chakravarty T, Mathur M, Holzhey D, Pershad A, Fang HK, O'Hair D, Jones N, Mahadevan VS, Dumonteil N, Rodés-Cabau J, Piazza N, Ferrari E, Ciaburri D, Nejjari M, DeLago A, Sorajja P, Zahr

F, Rajagopal V, Whisenant B, Shah PB, Sinning JM, Witkowski A, Eltchaninoff H, Dvir D, Martin B, Attizzani GF, Gaia D, Nunes NSV, Fassa AA, Kerendi F, Pavlides G, Iyer V, Kaddissi G, Witzke C, Wudel J, Mishkel, Raybuck B, Wang C, Waksman R, Palacios I, Crib-ier A, Webb J, Bapat V, Reisman M, Makkar R, Leon M, Rihal C, Vahanian A, O'Neill W, Feldman T. 1-year outcomes of transcatheter mitral valve replacement in patients with severe mitral annular calcification. *J Am Coll Cardiol* 2018;71:1841–1853.

Mitral stenosis produced by infective endocarditis involving a previously anatomically normal valve

Charles S. Roberts, MD[a], Gregory P. Milligan, MD, MPH[b], Robert C. Stoler, MD[b], Paul A. Grayburn, MD[b], and William C. Roberts, MD[b]

[a]Department of Cardiac Surgery, Baylor University Medical Center and the Baylor Scott & White Heart and Vascular Hospital, Dallas, Texas; [b]Division of Cardiology, Department of Internal Medicine, Baylor University Medical Center and the Baylor Scott & White Heart and Vascular Hospital, Dallas, Texas

ABSTRACT

Described herein is a 63-year-old man who developed methicillin-sensitive *Staphylococcus aureus* endocarditis on a previously anatomically normal mitral valve. The resulting vegetations were so large that severe mitral stenosis resulted. The development of valve stenosis due exclusively to infective endocarditis is extremely rare.

KEYWORDS Cerebral emboli; infective endocarditis; mitral stenosis; mitral valve replacement

nfective endocarditis (IE) most commonly attacks a previously anatomically normal valve or one previously mildly deformed (e.g., bicuspid aortic valve, mitral valve prolapse) but one functioning normally or causing only mild regurgitation.[1–3] In this scenario, the superimposed IE usually causes some regurgitation or worsens that already present. IE superimposed on a previously stenotic valve is uncommon. The vegetations of IE may cause no dysfunction or, if they do, the result is usually pure regurgitation.[2] IE by itself causing valvular stenosis is rare.[4–8] Such was the case, however, in the patient described herein.

CASE DESCRIPTION

A 63-year-old man was known to have systemic hypertension, diabetes mellitus, chronic obstructive pulmonary disease, abdominal aortic aneurysm (3.5 cm), and obesity (body mass index 33 kg/m^2). At the age of 54 years, chest pain prompted percutaneous coronary intervention, which was repeated in 2017. In early September 2018, he underwent left leg femoral artery angioplasty. Several days later, he noticed a lump in the left groin, the insertion site for his peripheral arterial procedure, followed shortly by fever, nausea, vomiting, and hypotension prompting admission to Baylor University Medical Center. Culture of the groin "lump" grew methicillin-sensitive *Staphylococcus aureus*, and he was treated with nafcillin. There was no precordial murmur. The lungs were clear to auscultation. Echocardiogram 2 days after hospitalization disclosed a mass in the mitral orifice attached to the mitral leaflets, causing an estimated 8 mm Hg mean transvalvular gradient *(Figure 1)*. Repeat echocardiogram 20 days later showed the mitral mass had increased in size, and the estimated mean transmitted gradient had increased to 14 mm Hg *(Figure 1)*.

Mitral valve replacement was performed 2 days after the last echocardiogram. The large intramitral mass was excised as well as debris in the mitral annular area (ring abscess) *(Figure 2)*. Because of ring abscess just caudal to the aortic valve, its three cusps, each devoid of vegetation, were also excised. His postoperative course was uneventful, and he was asymptomatic when contacted a year after the cardiac valve operation.

DISCUSSION

The first report describing valvular stenosis produced by a large vegetation appeared in 1967.[4] Subsequently, several additional cases of valvular stenosis produced by IE on previously nonstenotic cardiac valves have been reported.[5–8] As in all prior reports, the cause of the mitral stenosis in our patient was due entirely to the large vegetation obstructing mitral inflow into the left ventricle.

Relatively little data is available on the relation of vegetation size to outcome. Leitman and colleagues[9] described 50

Corresponding author: Charles S. Roberts, MD, 621 N. Hall Street, Suite 120, Dallas, TX 75226 (e-mail: Charles.Roberts@BSWHealth.org)

Color versions of one or more of the figures in the article can be found online at www.tandfonline.com/ubmc.

Received May 1, 2019; Accepted May 7, 2019.

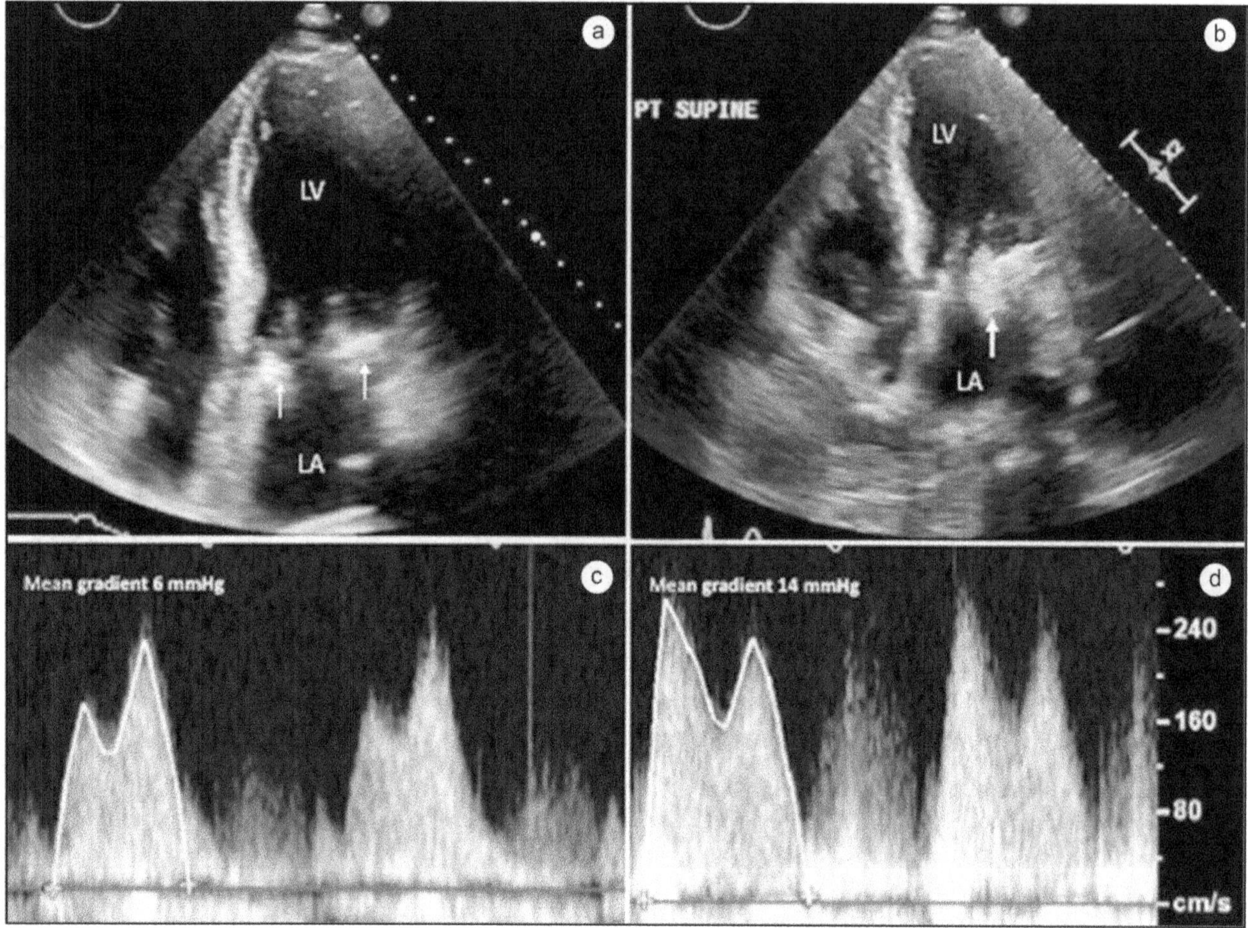

Figure 1. Four-chamber views from **(a)** initial study and **(b)** 1 month later. Mitral annular calcium (arrows) is present on the initial study, with no evidence of endocarditis. A large vegetation (large arrow) is seen 1 month later. **(c)** Continuous wave Doppler of mitral inflow showing a mean gradient of 6 mm Hg on initial study, **(d)** which increased to 14 mm Hg due to obstruction from the large vegetation.

patients with IE involving native mitral valves and 34 involving native aortic valves. Although the reasons are not entirely clear, vegetations ≥ 1 cm, type of causative microorganism (specifically *Staphylococcus* sp.), and age >60 years appeared to worsen prognosis (increased need for operation and increased mortality).

Relatively little information also is available on the relation of vegetation size to antibiotic(s) used to treat the IE. Rohmann and colleagues[10] studied 183 patients with IE by transesophageal echocardiogram and found vegetations on the native mitral valve alone in 89, on the aortic valve alone in 134, and on both valves in 40. The patients were followed from 2 to 186 weeks (mean 76). The initial vegetation size (8.4 ± 1.3 mm) fell with antibiotic therapy (to 7.8 ± 1.4 mm) in the group in whom an organism was isolated. Late follow-up (30 weeks) showed considerable further loss of vegetation size or total loss of the vegetation. The authors found that different antibiotics had different effects on vegetation size: vancomycin-associated treatment was related to a 45% reduction, penicillin-resistant drugs to a 15% increase, and cephalosporin to a 40% increase in vegetation size. None of

the patients described by Leitman et al or by Rohmann et al appeared to have developed valvular stenosis.

1. Arnett EA, Roberts WC. Active infective endocarditis: a clinicopathologic analysis of 137 necropsy patients. *Curr Probl Cardiol.* 1976;1(7): 1–75. doi:10.1016/0146-2806(76)90003-7.

2. Roberts WC, Oluwole BO, Fernicola DJ. Comparison of active infective endocarditis involving a previously stenotic versus a previously nonstenotic aortic valve. *Am J Cardiol.* 1993;71(12):1082–1088. doi:10.1016/0002-9149(93)90577-Y.

3. Fernicola DJ, Roberts WC. Clinicopathologic features of active infective endocarditis isolated to the mitral valve. *Am J Cardiol.* 1993; 71(13):1186–1197. doi:10.1016/0002-9149(93)90644-R.

4. Roberts WC, Ewy GA, Glancy DL, Marcus FI. Valvular stenosis produced by active infective endocarditis. *Circulation.* 1967;36(3): 449–451. doi:10.1161/01.CIR.36.3.449.

5. Sach PV, Laker JB, Barlow JB. Severe aortic stenosis produced by bacterial endocarditis. *BMJ.* 1969;3:97–98. doi:10.1136/bmj.3.5662.97.

6. Copeland JG, Salomon NW, Steinson EB, Popp RL, Shumway NE. Acute mitral valve obstruction from infective endocarditis. *J Thorac Cardiovasc Surg.* 1979;78:28–30.

7. Davies MK, Ireland MA, Clarke DB. Infective endocarditis from group C streptococci causing stenosis of both the aortic and mitral valves. *Thorax.* 1981;36(1):69–71. doi:10.1136/thx.36.1.69.

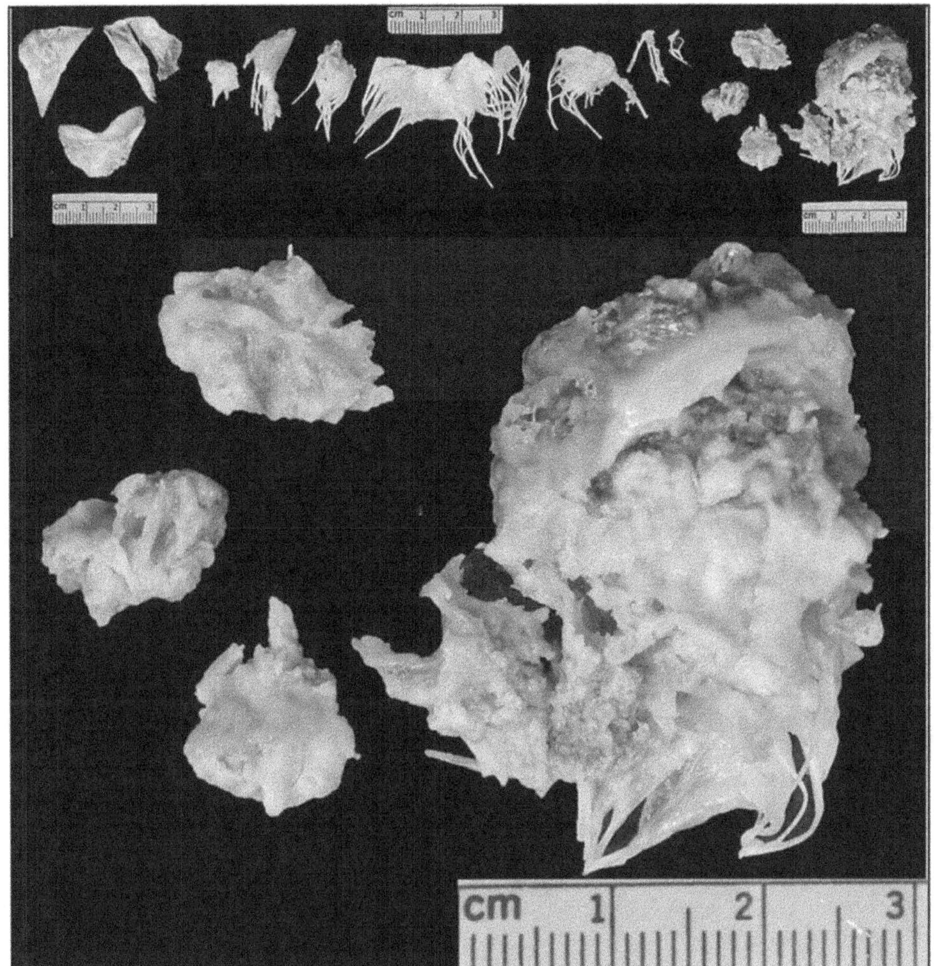

Figure 2. Photographs of the entire operatively excised mitral valve (top) and close-up of the vegetation obstructing the mitral orifice. Scattered microorganisms, foci of polymorphonuclear and mononuclear cells, large collections of fibrin, and a few small calcific fragments were present histologically in the large vegetation.

8. Hart MA, Shroff GR. Infective endocarditis causing mitral valve stenosis: a rare but deadly complication: a case report. *J Med Case Reports* 2017;11:44.

9. Leitman M, Dreznik Y, Tyomkin V, Fuchs T, Krakover R, Vered Z. Vegetation size in patients with infective endocarditis. *Eur Heart J Cardiovasc Imag.* 2012;13(4):330–338.

10. Rohmann S, Erbel R, Darius H, Makowski T, Meyer J. Effect of antibiotic treatment on vegetation size and complication rate in infective endocarditis. *Clin Cardiol.* 1997;20(2): 132–140.